The Shunt Brothers

A TRUE STORY

DOREEN KAY KAINE

The Shunt Brothers

A True Story

Doreen Kay Kaine

Table of Contents

Part Three: Another Difficult Journey

Part Four: Co-existing Conditions in the Shunt Brothers

Part Five: The Shunt Brothers Share Their CT's and MRI's

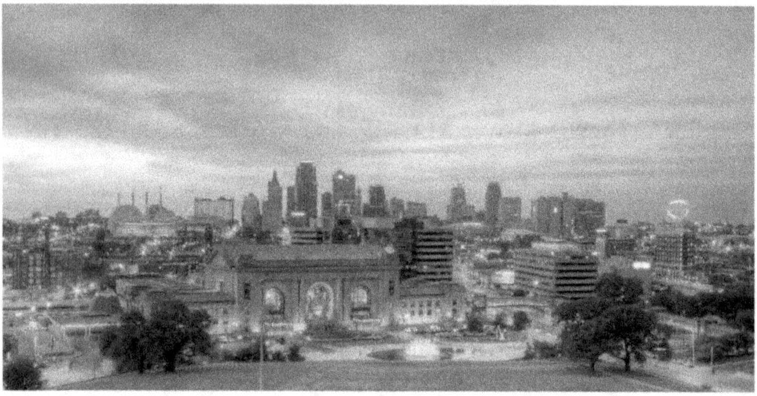

Introduction

I am writing this book to shed light on a neurological condition that is hopelessly misdiagnosed to this day. The condition has an odd name, Normal Pressure Hydrocephalus.

The lucky ones get the correct diagnosis and can go on to live productive lives. Those misdiagnosed are doomed to a life of cognitive decline, unsteadiness on their feet leading to frequent falls, tiny shuffling steps, and urinary issues. Most likely they will end up in a nursing home with a diagnosis of dementia. There are numerous types of dementia with similar and overlapping symptoms: frontal lobe, Lewy body, Alzheimer's, and vascular dementia. So NPH is easily mixed up with a misdiagnosis of dementia. Also, many of the movement disorders in NPH mimic Parkinson's disease. Without treatment it is impossible to get better, only worse. It is estimated that 10 percent of any nursing home population is suffering from this undiagnosed condition. Maybe one of your loved ones could be helped with the correct diagnosis. That is my goal in writing this book.

Medical professionals think this condition is "rare" and are very reluctant to even test for it. They will also discount the possibility that it could be inherited, although there is ongoing research on the genetic component. This is readily available to anyone who has Google or another search engine. Apparently, this possibility is never taught in medical schools. I am not writing this saga to bash the medical profession. Just wanting to shed light on a condition that is woefully misdiagnosed. I am not a medical professional, just someone who lived through this nightmare.

It is also a personal story of the man I married in 1978 and his family. He was born into a family of five boys in Kansas City, Missouri. They resided just across State Line Road that straddles Missouri and Kansas. Their father came down with this mysterious condition in 1980 and somehow got the right diagnosis and treatment. My husband served in Vietnam in the late 60s and came home with PTSD and later developed the symptoms of this disease. But it took years of going to Kansas City Veteran's Hospital, outside neurologists (a whopping seven in all) to get a diagnosis. It was frustrating and unbelievably stressful. Then in the past few years not one but three of my husband's brothers started showing signs of the same disease. By keeping in touch with their wives and one daughter they were all treated as well. Now tell me it can't be inherited?

I will be relying on medical records and physician notes to tell their story. I will not name any physician or try to embarrass anyone. I will name the hospitals they went to because it was an important part of the story. Most are in Kansas City, but we did travel to Mayo Clinic in Rochester, Minnesota and one brother was treated in St. Louis. My medical research will be cited and can be verified on Google, PubMed and NIH. The Hydrocephalus Association estimates that nearly 700,000 adults have Normal Pressure Hydrocephalus, but it is often misdiagnosed as Alzheimer's or Parkinson's disease. In fact by various accounts, only between less than 7 to up to 20 percent of the people with the disease are accurately diagnosed. I think the misdiagnosed make up a large number of our elderly, especially those confined to nursing homes.

If this book can reach a fraction of them, it will be worth it. Of course, the caretakers, the husbands and wives and daughters and sons must take the lead and question their medical providers and if you are turned away then seek that second, third, or fourth opinion. Let the journey begin!

Part 1

The History of the Shunt Brothers

This is a story about how eventually five out of six family members were diagnosed and received shunts for NPH. Their father Ray Sr. in 1980, my husband Tim in 2014, then his brother Pat in 2021, and Ray Jr. and Clancy in 2024. I don't think a single doctor brought up or believed the possibility of heredity causing this horrific disease. I don't believe they have identified the specific genetic factor that could cause this, but they do have possibilities and sounds like more research is needed. Maybe then we wouldn't be told again and again that it can't be inherited. One can only hope. It certainly was a learning journey for me as I had no idea other families have been identified all over the world and there is a good amount of research into the genetic component. Perhaps the only ones who are not aware of this research are the practicing doctors who routinely misdiagnose this disease and discount or ignore heredity. Hopefully this book will help in some way!

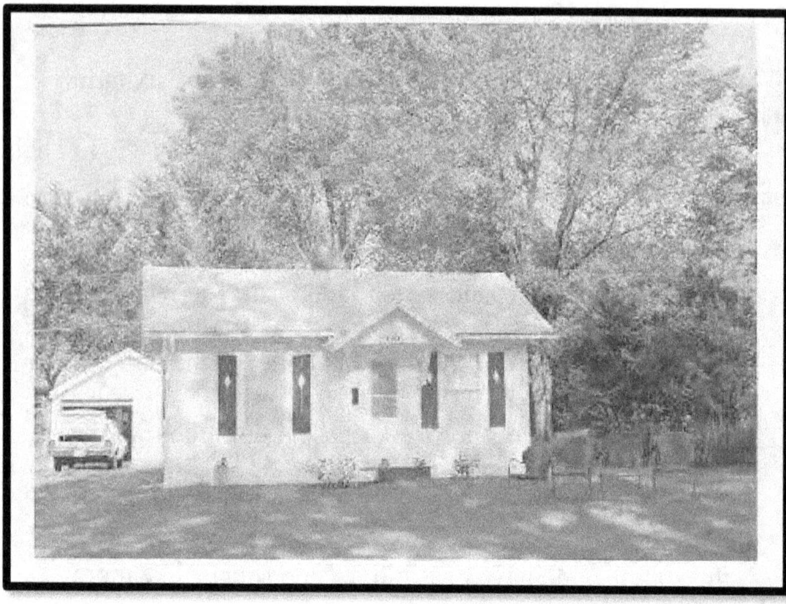

HOME SWEET HOME

1

This is the small white framed house with cheery red shutters and matching lawn chairs where all the brothers grew up. It consisted of a front room, back room, tiny kitchen, small bathroom and a bedroom. The boys slept in the back room and on a pullout couch in the front room. Space was tight in this tiny house.

Dad worked for the Kansas City Board of Education and delivered supplies to all the public schools. He also was a fantastic book binder at the Kansas City Public Library. Mom stayed at home raising five boys but also took in ironing because money was tight. They went to church religiously and were all raised in the Christian faith. Mom cooked delicious meals every day which always included a freshly made dessert. Guess what? There were never any leftovers with five hungry boys.

In the late 70s their Dad began having some strange symptoms. The next to the oldest son Casey has agreed to share his recollection of what happened to him and how he got help. He was the first one in the family to get a shunt after their primary care physician diagnosed him with NPH.

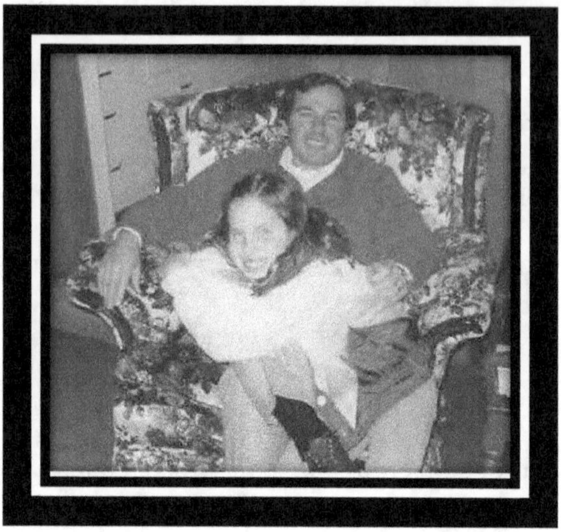

Casey's Recollection

2

Our family's first encounter with NPH was approximately 1980 when my father was 70 years old. This was when I, along with my two children, stopped by my parent's house after sledding. Sadly, my father was slumped down into an easy chair, as if he had a stroke. This was the early diagnosis and probably would have remained the diagnosis except for my parent's primary care physician. Their doctor doggedly stayed after the search to find the underlying cause of what was going on with my dad's condition.

It took a week of digging, but in the end NPH was the diagnosis and a shunt was put in. The results were immediate and miraculous. No more paralysis or lack of speech. His old life and vitality were back. He was restored. He died when he was 89 in 1999. Long before social media, the Shunt Brothers patriarch was making his beliefs known by putting signs on his car. Here is one of them:

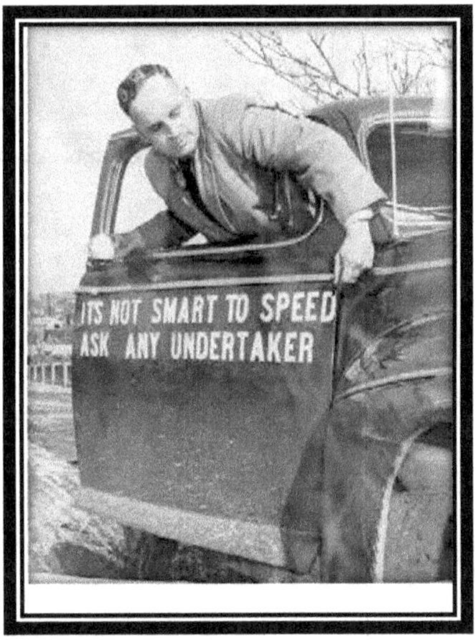

Tim's Long Journey

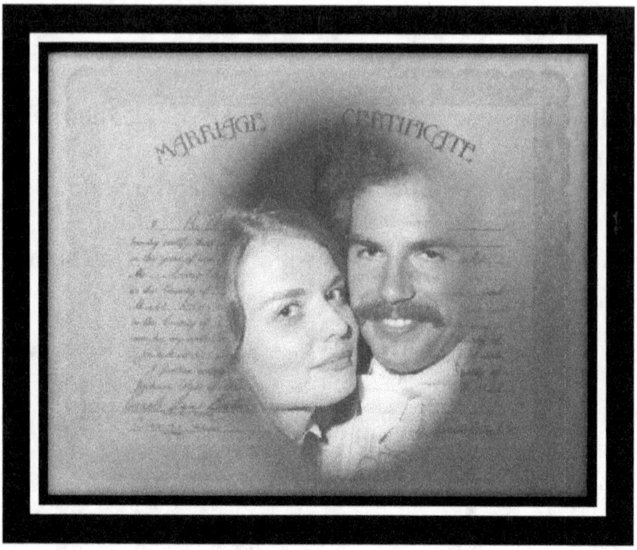

I married that handsome guy on the left in August of 1978. Tim was the only brother to serve in Vietnam and returned with a bad case of posttraumatic stress disorder. I could write another book on those years dealing with that condition, but this one will only focus on getting the diagnosis and treatment of NPH.

I'm not exactly positive when Tim's symptoms began but I am going to rely on records from Kansas City Veteran's

Hospital. They put him through numerous tests over the years and I will not name any doctors but I will put their comments in quotes so you will know that's who I am quoting. It seems he had every test imaginable and went through a plethora of probable diagnoses, but all proved to be wrong.

I became a Google warrior and started doing my own research. Lots of it. I came across a well-respected kidney specialist who developed the symptoms of NPH but could not get anyone to listen to him or treat him. As he finally overcame the system and got the surgery he needed and a shunt implanted, it dawned on me that those same symptoms were what my husband was going through. Could it be related to what his dad had so many years ago? Possibly.

- But I digress and will go back to KCVA and their attempts to diagnose these baffling symptoms my husband was having. They have been described as Wet, Wacky, and Wobbly. I don't like that nomenclature and won't use it because I think it's an unkind description of people who are suffering.

KCVA Medical Records:

I believe the walking difficulties were the first sign things were not right. Tim also became very unbalanced and fell numerous times. They called it "ataxia." The gait problems were maybe vascular in nature or neurological issues they thought. So, he went through testing for both. Tim was also having cognitive difficulties, memory problems, etc. This testing was done the same year, and those results are included.

Aug. 21,2013

"Reviewed patients CTA in vascular conference today. His CTA is clean without evidence of any significant vascular occlusion to explain his symptoms. No indication for

vascular intervention. Defer work up and treatment to primary care physician."

Aug.26, 2013-

" Wife states that he had an EMG/NCS at outside facility and it was negative."

Sept 5, 2013-

"This patient reports that the leg weakness began in 2012. He states that the weakness is equal in both legs. He describes pain in both legs below the knees after he first stands after a prolonged period of sitting. He states that the pain is so great that it immobilizes him at times and does occur intermittently while sitting. Any movement, not just walking, aggravates the leg pain. When it does occur with walking, it is relieved with resting a few times."

We had just returned from Nashville, Tennessee to celebrate our 35th wedding anniversary that year. Not a good idea. Tim had to walk a great deal and was in tremendous pain. We went on several sightseeing tours, and he would just plop on the floor to alleviate the pain. People began scrambling for chairs to try and help him. Going to a concert at Ryman Auditorium he did nothing but close his eyes and say he felt sick. I was becoming desperate for some answers. And Primary Care did not have them. Defer indeed! It would be another full year before we had any answers.

Next, we will discuss declining cognitive abilities. Tim took numerous batteries of the most common dementia screening tests. These were performed at the KCVA hospital, but he was also thoroughly screened at Mayo Clinic. I will include excerpts from both facilities.

Dec 13, 2004- KCVA

"Neuropsychological testing was done, and it was found: The results indicative of a person who is having problems with attention and concentration, which may be due to his current psychiatric condition rather than to an organic cognitive dysfunction, at this time. Overall, the results of the neuropsychological evaluation fall within borderline."

9+Feb.20,2013

"Efficient mental flexibility as measured by a rapid visual motor scanning task was rated as severely impaired.

This represents a significant decline compared to his prior average ability to complete this task within expected time limits.

There was evidence of moderate cognitive impairment across a number of abilities. Similar to his prior exams, he continued to display a pattern of deficits in attention and immediate memory, However, there also appears to have been a general decline in cognitive functioning compared to his two prior exams."

I will briefly touch on urinary issues as it is not a favorite topic of conversation, but it also was a symptom. This one was also a little complicated as Tim had prostate cancer and had a prostectomy in 2013. So urinary incontinence and urgency were noted both pre-op and post-op but also seemed to be a symptom of NPH. I won't include any doctor's notes, but it definitely was an issue.

Misdiagnoses and the Whopping Seven Neurologists in 2014

This was most definitely a miserable year as I was chasing an elusive diagnosis for Tim that I was fairly sure I had already figured out. I had folders of research and carried Tim's medical records wherever we went. He was getting increasingly irritable and hard to deal with in the car as we made our rounds. We ended up going to most of the major hospitals in the Kansas City area: St. Luke's East in Lee's Summit, KU Medical Center in Kansas City, Kansas, Research Hospital in Kansas City, Centerpoint Hospital in Independence, Kansas City Veteran's Hospital in Kansas City, Mo. And finally, Mayo Clinic in Rochester, Minnesota. Two trips there but it was totally worth it.

Many just said it was a complicated case and they were reluctant to make any diagnosis. Among the wrong ones were:

Frontal lobe dementia

Alzheimer's

Parkinson's Disease

Dementia (unspecified)

The only one who brought up normal pressure hydrocephalus was a Patient Advocate who whispered it in the ear of the neurologist at KU. I overheard it so we discussed the possibility of it being this disease. Tim was so anxious on this visit; he was pacing outside the office door and wouldn't come in to sit down. So, the neurologist said she could do a spinal tap but was afraid he wouldn't lie still for the procedure. So that was as far as we got, and we drove home.

It was a neurosurgeon at Centerpoint who finally agreed to see us and would try to help. When he came out of his office after reviewing the latest CT scan, he said it showed excess fluid and although he couldn't guarantee good outcomes, he was willing to consider a Ventriculoperitoneal shunt. But that would depend on the results of a lumbar puncture which he was willing to do. Hallelujah!

So, Tim had the spinal tap done on October 31, 2014. Then we anxiously awaited the results. I was not sure they followed the recommended procedure as there were no cognitive tests before or after. They did check his wide-based gait, but the physical therapist was over an hour late to check for improvement. But I noticed a vast improvement and at home Tim kept talking and saying how good he felt. He said it felt like "a load had been lifted from my brain."

So, we waited. I was able to get into Mayo Clinic in Rochester, Minnesota on November 13, 2014, so we jumped in the car and drove six hours to get there.

If there is some doubt about the improvement shown after a spinal tap, ask for the ELD which stands for External Lumbar

Drainage. They drain a small amount of CSF every day and look for improvement in a 3 day time period. Also many people report no real improvement from the spinal tap, but they do have the symptoms and do benefit from shunting.

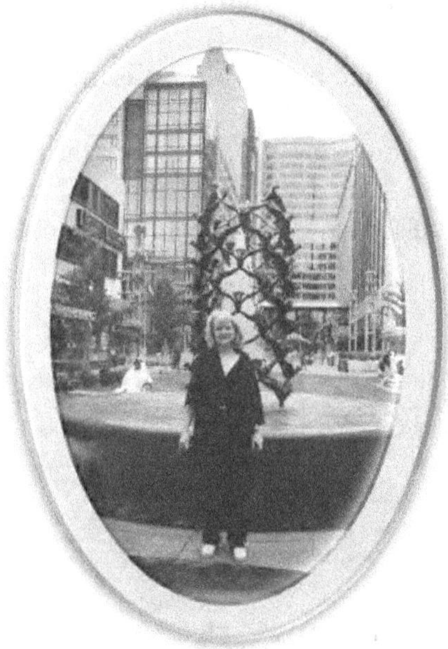

I am a native of Minnesota, having been born in the small town of Slayton in the southwest corner of the state. We lived on a farm with our grandparents and raised chickens and cows and probably other livestock too. We moved to Kansas City when I was four years old. So, when I cross the Minnesota state line, I kind of feel like I am home. I love looking at the crops that go as far as the eye can see. Brings back good memories.

But we were here to get some answers and confirmation of what my husband had been fighting for several years. With the spinal tap done and no actual results or surgery scheduled, I was hoping for some confirmation from the doctors at Mayo. Again, their notes are in bold type and have not been altered.

Nov. 13,2014-Mayo Clinic

"The patient is a 66-year-old right-handed gentleman with progressive difficulties with walking and cognition. His cognitive profile shows significant abnormalities. He has a previous Pet scan of his brain that showed diffuse abnormalities. He has also developed some atrophy in the frontal lobes. There is a family history of normal pressure hydrocephalus. I think given the improvement after the

large volume tap; it would be useful to proceed with the ventriculoperitoneal shunt. We will plan to see the patient back in six months' time after he has hopefully had the shunt. If they refuse to do the shunt closer to home, we could consider having a large volume lumbar puncture here and an evaluation with our neurosurgeons here."

<u>Diagnoses</u>

#1 Cognitive Difficulties

#2 Gait Difficulties

#3 Possible Normal Pressure Hydrocephalus

#4 Urine Incontinence

After over two years of searching for answers, WE FINALLY HAD A DIAGNOSIS!!!

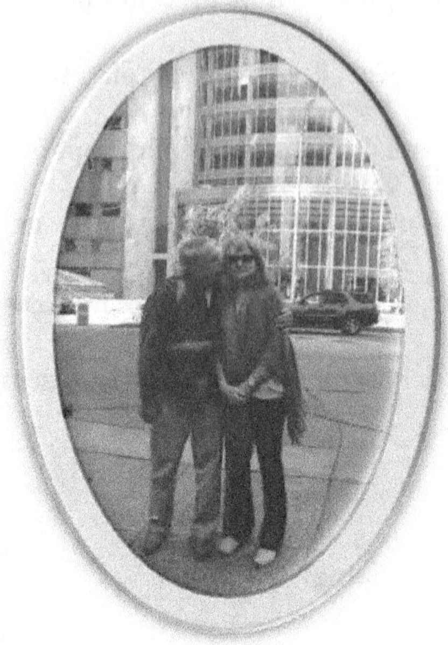

THANK YOU MAYO CLINIC!!!

After returning home, the surgery was performed at Centerpoint Hospital in Independence, Mo. on December 18, 2014. After reading his notes this neurosurgeon sounded like he was still unsure of the success of the lumbar puncture and would have continued to delay any surgery. But after I shared Mayo's diagnosis, he changed his mind.

Postscript: This neurosurgeon also made a big mistake with the surgery, and it had to be revised in May. He didn't get the catheter that drains the fluid in the ventricle, so it was basically not draining at all. This was not discovered for 5 months, so Tim's recovery was put on hold for those months. If I said everyone lived happily ever after the shunt was implanted, I would be lying. They do alleviate some of the worst symptoms like the shuffling walk, urinary incontinence, and foggy thinking. But depending on how long the condition has been untreated, many cognitive issues remain because the brain has been damaged. Tim suffered a stroke in May 2016 and that brought its own complications. Is it worth it to have it? Undoubtedly, there are many miraculous stories out there.

- I have asked Tim's three brothers to tell their own stories of their symptoms, diagnosis and shunt surgeries. Then I will share the thread that their wives and daughter kept while they were being diagnosed. It helps a lot to have family support during these times.

Lessons Learned

4

1. **You must be the voice for the person who is suffering from this disease. You must speak up to the doctors and advocate for them. It does no good to be quiet or submissive. We are taught that doctors always know best, but with this condition that is not always the case.**
2. **It doesn't hurt to have some basic knowledge of what NPH looks like on a CT or MRI. I always ask to see the CT and have it explained to me. Most doctors will do that. Then have a copy made so you can keep it for reference and comparison.**
3. **If they do a CT scan and say they do not have Normal Pressure Hydrocephalus then ask for a lumbar puncture. This is noninvasive and not that difficult to do. Mistakes are made on reading NPH on CT scans. MRIs are better. Ask for one if**

possible. My husband couldn't have one because of a pacemaker.

4. **If you ask them if this condition is inherited, they will almost inevitably say no. There is a body of research that proves otherwise. I will share some of this at the end of the book.**

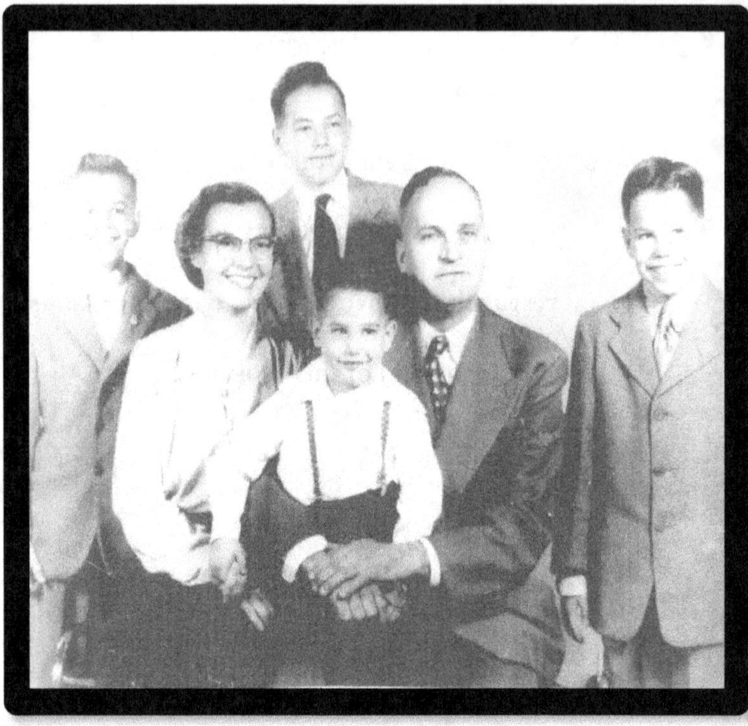

It is difficult to find a picture with all five brothers. One always seems to be missing. So, I will share the young boy's picture and then grown-up boy's picture later. Handsome boys aren't they? From left to right we have Pat, Casey, and Tim. In front, we have Mom and Dad and the baby of the family, Clancy.

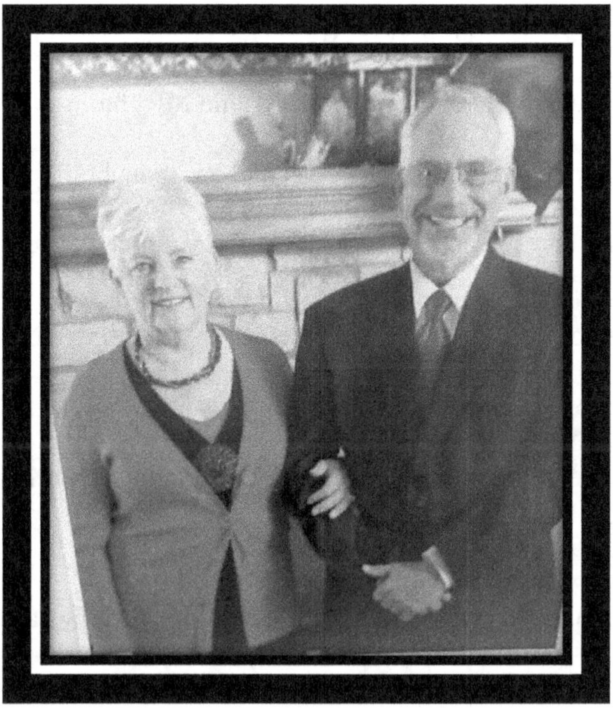

Pat's Story

(as told by his wife, Kathy)

5

Several years prior to getting bad, he kept complaining about his memory. His regular Doctor referred him to a neurologist because Pat was worried about his memory issues. He did the testing, and said he didn't see any abnormalities. The neurologist did not discuss NPH. He then referred him to a psychologist. He did some tests CT and MRI but wanted to refer him to another psychologist and Pat thought they were wasting his time and money, so he never returned to see them.

In May of 2021 his symptoms seemed to be getting worse and closer together. He couldn't pick up his feet to walk, therefore falling more frequently. He thought he was losing control of his bladder. He had bouts of anger, (due to the issues that he was having and not knowing what the cause was.)

I was sitting watching TV one evening and it came to mind that his father and his brother had gone through the same thing. I called my sister-in-law Doreen and visited with her concerning his brother. She walked me through all the symptoms and what had to be done to correct all of the issues. I called the next day to his regular doctor, and took him within a couple of days. The doctor gave him a referral to a neurosurgeon. On June 2, 2021 he went for his first visit with this neurosurgeon. He reviewed the CT and MRI at length that had been performed in the last few months. His assessment and plan were as follows:

From the neurosurgeon's report:

"The patient does have evidence of a combination of brain atrophy and ventriculomegaly. Especially on the coronal images of the MRI, the ventriculomegaly does appear to be somewhat out of proportion to the atrophy. In this regards, he does have evidence of normal pressure hydrocephalus, although he may also be suffering from degenerative brain issues. His gait is very slow and shuffling, so Parkinson's is always a potential consideration. His bladder control issue is just a small amount of dribbling that occurs at night if he cannot get to the bathroom in time. He does have other family members that have done well with shunts. The family is

considering a VP shunt in his case. We discussed the potential surgical risks and benefits in length. They do understand that over drainage can be an issue along with shunt malfunction or infection, etc. The risk of subdural hematoma/hygroma."

He then referred him to the neurologist, stating that he needed to schedule him as soon as possible.

Note to provider:

"Please evaluate for memory difficulties, mild incontinence and gait problems. Our question is whether or not this is dementia with any degree of Parkinson's or if it is a more clear-cut normal pressure hydrocephalus."

His first visit with the neurologist was on 6-10-21. He went over all his medical information. After review, he said he wanted to proceed with the testing of NPH. On 6-21-21 he went to have his testing done. They tested his gait and his ability to get up and down to a chair. He was then taken back to have a spinal tap done. When he was done with the spinal tap, they brought him back and repeated the testing that was done prior to the spinal tap. He then referred him back to the neurosurgeon who scheduled the surgery to put the shunt in. The surgery was done on 7-26-21. He stayed overnight and was discharged on 7-27-21.

The week of August 2021 he had issues with pain and nausea. We went back to the neurosurgeon and it was determined that the drain tube was inserted into the muscle of the stomach.

He had to undergo surgery to get the drain tube in the right place and draining in the stomach.

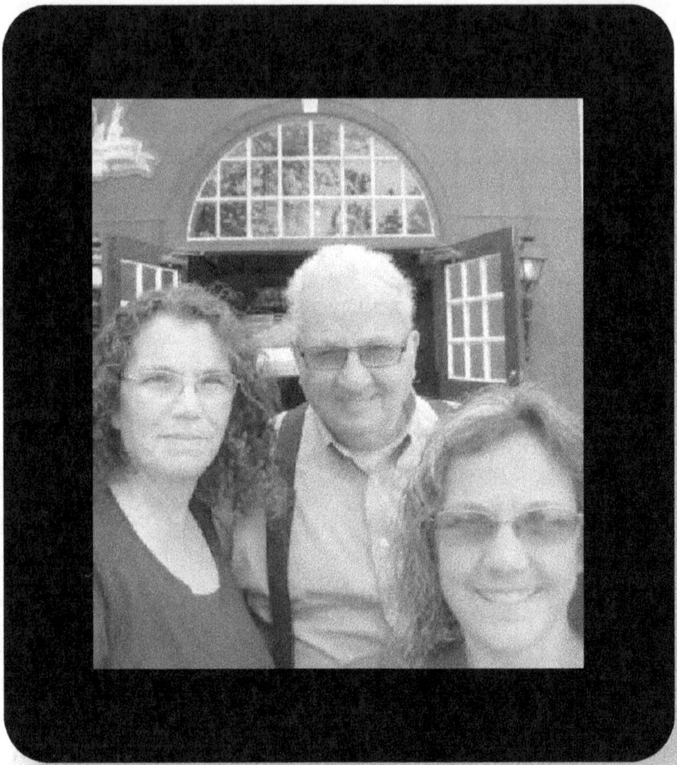

Ray Jr's Story

(as told by his daughter Marsha)

6

First and foremost, before I share my father's journey, I'd like to thank our Lord Jesus Christ for my aunt, this opportunity, travel mercies and my dad's amazing doctor. My aunt is the family pioneer of our idiopathic Normal Pressure Hydrocephalus experiences with her research skills, sharing her knowledge and encouraging us to not give up. Her husband, my uncle, was the first of this second generation to be diagnosed. She has suggested we get a second opinion or third opinion until we get a correct diagnosis. We have traveled many miles and up to eight hours across several state lines for tests, diagnosis, surgeries and follow-up care.

It is my hope, that while sharing this extremely rare family and my father's journey, you will be encouraged or even validated. Please take my family experiences seriously and use them as a roadmap to help you along the way in getting your loved one or friend diagnosed and treated. I hope this book will shed light on a very important yet very misdiagnosed complex medical condition.

We have been ignored, misinformed and even told that we are wrong. They emphatically told us that this is not an inherited condition. Just as I told my aunt, I will never be convinced of that now with two generations and five out of six immediate family members having it. Yes I am curious, concerned and have questions as my generation is next in line. The average age for NPH diagnosis is sixty and we are at the brink. Will any of my cousins or myself have it? My grandfather had five sons so is there a gender factor?

My family first learned about Normal Pressure Hydrocephalus when my grandfather was diagnosed with it in 1980. He lived with a shunt for 19 years and passed away at the age of 89.

Of the five "boys" it was my uncle, the fourth born, who was diagnosed first. He was experiencing what we now know as the classic symptoms. It was no easy task to get a diagnosis. In fact it was a lengthy and difficult challenge. It was my aunt's perseverance and knowledge that finally got him diagnosed about 10 years ago at the age of 65. His story is in this book and his pioneer wife is the reason we are able to share with you.

Now to share my father's story. He is a retired Kansas City, Kansas fireman that lives in Illinois \where his wife's family is. It amazes me that at the current age of eighty four years he still lives at home and does many things for himself. I have a variety of work experience including UPS supervisor, office assistant among many other things but it is my past experience as a CNA Activity Leader in Memory Care and family experience that gives me familiarity with cognitive changes. While I cared deeply for my residents and patients, it's a whole new ball game when it's your family. I have noticed more changes over the past few years and questioned if it was "normal" for this stage of life. Even I have memory issues so why wouldn't he? Things really changed about four years ago. It was a bit difficult, on my part, to speak up too much when he is being cared for and lives four hours away. I greatly appreciate that he is being cared for, in his own home and not in a facility. He and his wife qualify for excellent benefits to help them with many everyday responsibilities. This includes their breakfast and lunch being fixed for them at home, daily dishes, laundry, floors, trash, groceries picked up, transportation to the doctor when needed and physical therapy, mostly at home, when needed.

When I brought him to Kansas City for visits, I could definitely see the changes and inconsistency with confusion and memory issues but I would answer his questions as if it were the first time asking. We tried a little notepad in his shirt pocket with our daily plan written down but oftentimes he didn't remember it was there. There were times of great clarity and detail then there was very little. Most would think it's beginning or intermediate Alzheimer's which is part of the complexity of getting NPH properly diagnosed. You must go on symptoms more than any test or scan. It's more than memory or confusion. They, oftentimes are off balance which causes falls, and have a strong urgency to urinate. With the inability to think clearly or walk very far or quickly, they have embarrassing accidents.

Since 2016 there were several trips, in Illinois, to the Emergency Department for not feeling right, confusion, weakness, heart problems and Covid-19 to name a few. On August 19, 2020 one of the helpers took him to Alton Memorial Hospital ER. His pulse was very low, he felt weak, and he was feeling bad. They needed to keep him for observation and more testing, but he could not take it any longer after 9 hours on a bed in a very noisy ER hallway. Being confused he thought they were not going to get to him for a few days and signed himself out.

June 1-7, 2022-Several falls occurred this week while the symptoms worsened.

June 9, 2022- About midnight of June 8-9 my dad apparently fell and did not have the ability to get off the floor and back into his bed. He was there for approximately five hours. Thankfully there were no bones broken and no serious injuries but how awful that must have been to not have the mental or physical ability to function. One of the scheduled helpers arrived that morning and ended up taking him to the ER. He was very weak and not feeling right. They arrived at OSF-Saint Anthony's Health Center which is near his home. While they were getting his information processed he was taken for a cat scan of his head. In the meantime they realized that his insurance was not accepted at this location. While the CT had already been done, they were not able to do anything else. He was released and taken home. A very IMPORTANT note here is that, call it what you will, he was "mistakenly" at the "wrong location" but they actually reported on his abnormal CT stating, "normal pressure hydrocephalus should be entertained in the appropriate clinical context." Amongst all the other medical terminology and jargon, it is this one sentence that was the first acknowledgment that he could have NPH as we had suspected with the family history. Unfortunately, I was not aware of this until much later.

His symptoms continued and worsened on this day to the point that he was incapacitated. He was then transported to Alton Memorial Hospital where his insurance is accepted. It was about the same time I was getting off work, in Kansas, when I was informed of his situation. I went to my house, quickly threw a bag together, went to fill up my car and drove four hours straight to the hospital where he was still in the ER. After being admitted, and several tests run, we learned he had Covid-19. I believed his condition was not caused by Covid. I stayed with my dad all day, every day of that week in the hospital. He could hardly walk, had a hard time with words, memory, was dizzy, off balance, and urgency to urinate was off the chart. A lot of difficulties were experienced but I'm grateful I was there and able to help him through it. As I monitored behaviors that week, I strongly felt he was experiencing more than Covid or normal aging. If only I had known about the abnormal CT that very same morning.

After two other hospital stays, they sent him to a nursing home for rehab which was not the answer. I went back to Illinois and quickly got him out. This was not what he needed. He was happy to be back home. They were sending two types of therapy to the house but it still was not the answer. I wanted a different doctor because this was way more than Covid. His symptoms of falling, being off balance, dizzy, headaches, memory, confusion, oftentimes his steps were reduced to tiny, shuffling steps and the urgency to urinate all continued.

August 2, 2022- Another ER visit and he was admitted to stay in the hospital. He was referred to a neurologist. Maybe he could finally get some help and we could get answers.

August 5, 2022- Office visit to his referred neurologist. Unfortunately this doctor did not listen and said it was basically normal aging. Follow-up visit with this doctor but he, flat out, would not listen to the family history or discuss the possibility of NPH. The doctor ignored and dismissed it so my dad's stepdaughter and husband got up, walked out, and never returned to him.

February 19, 2023- I brought my dad to town for a few days. It was always filled with getting his favorite BBQ ribs and visiting family and friends. This particular day, I had taken him to see one of his best, longtime friends, who had turned 92. We were visiting over some hot coffee at his kitchen table and enjoying the wildlife outside a large window. My dad got up to see something outside and he became off balanced and did what I call the sideways shuffle. He fell pretty hard and hurt his leg on the wooden chair. We decided it was getting evening time so he would stay the night in his friend's guestroom. I returned the next morning to get him and learned about his night. His friend found him in a rocking chair at 3:00 AM. My dad said he didn't know how to get out of it and back into the bed. His friend helped him, then returned to his room.

November 17, 2023-

He was not able to walk, felt terrible, could not comprehend how to get in the car, so again, he was taken by ambulance to the hospital where he stayed 5 days. He also had Covid again. By this time, I've been asking for another opinion, a new neurologist, answers and help. This was not Covid.

December 16-18, 2023-

We are never promised even another breath. I wanted the five brothers to have an opportunity to see each other and visit so I brought my dad to town for his side of the family Christmas dinner and get together. It was an amazing time, but we learned his youngest brother was diagnosed with a serious health condition. My dad used a walker and did pretty good during his visit but once he was back in Illinois things, once again, quickly took a turn and he was back in the hospital.

I had been communicating with my aunt quite a bit sharing updates on my dad's symptoms, what falls I knew about and several of his hospital visits. I started a chat thread so the four aunts could see the update with one post. By doing so, we learned that my youngest uncle was having the same symptoms. This chat thread has been invaluable. By sharing experiences, gaining knowledge and updates, he was able to get diagnosed with NPH about the same time as my father.

I was told that Illinois was at the bottom of the list for healthcare. I certainly could believe that after all of our frustrating dead-end experiences. We learned that his insurance was accepted in Missouri so I began trying to figure out how I could get my dad from Illinois and seen in Missouri. Was I to bring him to Kansas City, Missouri for doctor appointments and then back to Illinois? I didn't know but something had to be done and soon. He was declining and we needed answers.

December 20-27, 2023-Alton Memorial Hospital

Just a couple of days after his Kansas City visit, he was admitted for influenza, weakness, confusion and "altered mental status." The weakness was in both legs. The combination of confusion and weakness made walking a very difficult task. A walker was not much use at this point. Slow, tiny, shuffling steps for a short distance was about the best he could do. Oftentimes we had to use a wheelchair. Several more tests were run while he was there. Finally there was a doctor and a nurse who listened to our family history with NPH. Another CT was performed, a walking /gait test was done and the necessary lumbar puncture procedure was ordered. They drained a good amount of the excess fluid and finished the procedure. After resting, physical therapy came to repeat his walking exercise. There was a huge difference in his balance, understanding the instructions of where to walk, the walking speed, size of his steps, communication and memory. My dad was assigned a new neurosurgeon to follow-up with once he was released from the hospital. The new doctor was in St. Louis, Missouri, so that was huge to have an opportunity for care in Missouri.

January 1, 2024-Illinois
He had a fall in his kitchen but was able to get up with assistance and pulling on his wife's wheelchair.

January- 9.2024-

I was back in Illinois to attend our first appointment with the new neurosurgeon in his office. I wasn't sure what to think so

I looked up his information and shared it to my aunt's chat thread. There was positive feedback so I felt better. We got right in and had the best appointment. This doctor is FIRE! He is an expert in this field and things were explained to us, our questions were answered and surgery was set for two weeks. I was so relieved while being a bit nervous at the same time. It had been such a long journey of closed doors, then we were sitting in the office of the most qualified professional specialist.

January 21, 2024-

Watching the bad weather expected as I'm headed to Illinois for dad's surgery. Rain and ice across Kansas and Missouri. Babysitting went later than I expected so my start to Illinois was delayed until 2:00 PM. I made it safely.

January 22, 2024-

Freezing rain and a severe ice storm coated the city. Slipping and sliding, I put down ice melt to try and clear the way for my dad to safely get into the truck. His blood sugar was fantastic at 117, he had some cereal with limited medication and had a fall in the kitchen while trimming a thread on his pant cuff. I was able to break his fall so it was like slow motion and not as hard as it would have been. No serious injuries and got him up without any trouble. We managed to get dad safely into the truck. Just as we slowly pulled out of the drive and headed down the street, we received notice that surgery had been cancelled.

January 25, 2024-

After some delays, he was taken to the operating room at 3:45 PM. The surgery went really well with no complications so he did not have to go to ICU. He had inner sutures with outer staples. The CT shows the shunt is exactly where the doctor wants it. The setting is 1.5. It was a bit challenging through the night but I'm grateful I could stay on a sofa in his room and help him several times throughout the night.

My dad and his youngest brother received their shunts 3 weeks apart. We were in St. Louis, Missouri while his brother was in Kansas City, Kansas, 253 miles apart.

Our neurosurgeon, the expert, has said that he has never seen this situation where many family members have NPH.

January 26,2024-

Discharged from the hospital. I got him home and settled. We had a few trials finding the right medication for him but got him comfortable without the hard narcotics.

February 5, 2024-

I was back in Illinois and took him to his first post-surgery appointment. The doctor said things were looking great. He was impressed with his recovery and removed his staples. We discussed the shunt setting but did not change it.

February 6,2024-

Just twelve days after surgery and one day after staples removal. He was doing great so we planned on getting up early to go to the Missouri and Mississippi rivers to hopefully see some eagles. After removing the heavy frost from my car I helped him get in the car. We headed up the block for his favorite occasional morning treat- a cappuccino. I noticed someone coming up close behind me, so I turned and looked. There was my dad, no walker or cane, holding out a five dollar bill asking, "Do you want a doughnut Marsh?" A bit confused myself I answered "ummmmm Sure!" We went to the doughnut case as I looked around the aisle for his walker. I then looked up over the chip rack to see outside the window. There was my car, still running, but at least it didn't get stolen. It was a bit scary but I felt ecstatic at the same time. The difference that this caring doctor, surgery, and 12 days had made was astounding. Yes, we enjoyed our doughnut, cappuccino and saw some eagles. We even saw a nest with a couple young ones looking up over the edge.

April 8, 2024-

Visit to dad's and we shared the rare eclipse experience. He was doing great! I did some flower gardening for him which he was very happy about.

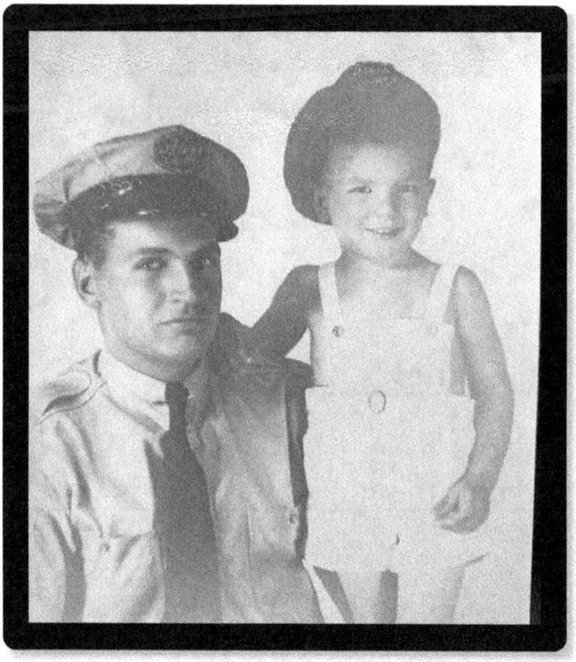

Ray Jr. at 3 years old with his father Ray Sr.

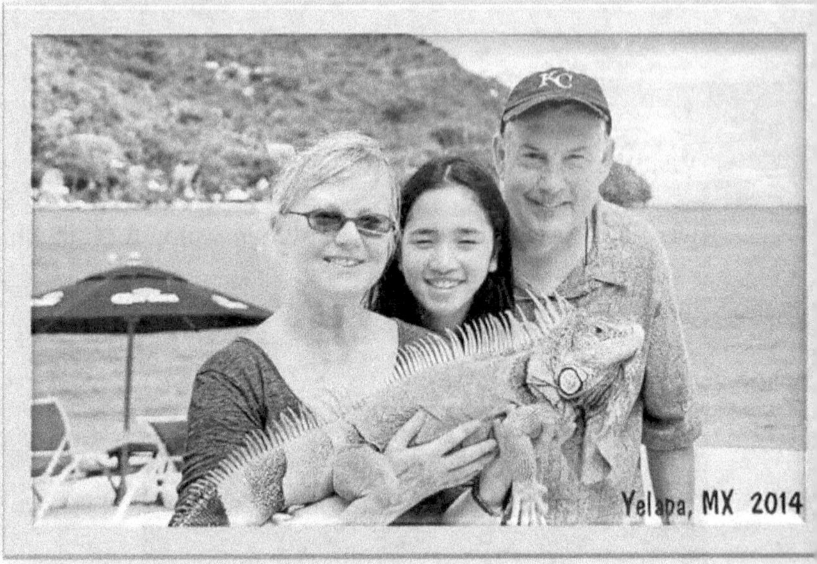

7

Clancy's story

Timeline and commentary by Ann, his wife

Clancy's recollection in bold type

2018- My earliest recollection of symptoms was probably when I started to have to shift weight from foot to foot. At first it wasn't too bad. But this was probably towards the

end of work when I was 66. It wasn't bad but it continued until the time I retired a couple years later. I was definitely not too steady standing still. And walking was OK.

2021- So then I retired. And by the summer I started doing stuff. I went to a podiatrist.

First episode:

July 3, 2022 -We drove to Kentucky for a 4-day trip on the Bourbon Trail, visiting some friends in Indiana on the way. We met them for dinner and Clancy seemed to have a bad reaction to the greasy fried fish when he came to bed that night. He didn't feel well and had difficulty getting into bed, seemed to lose control of his legs. This went on thru the night.

July 4, 2022- In the morning, he went for coffee, seemed a little better. We arrived in KY at the Airbnb, unloaded the car and took our luggage to the upstairs bedroom, which he managed with no problem. We had booked a river boat ride for that afternoon, and he seemed better so we continued our plans and boarded the boat. It was hot and I wondered why he was leaning on me uncomfortably on the boat. I kept nudging him but he didn't budge. At the end of the 1 hour boat ride, I was getting off the boat but Camilla, our daughter, and my cousin Jenny who had joined us for the trip, turned and saw that he couldn't move, and had to be helped off. Climbing the stairs from the dock took great effort. He headed to a porta-potty in the parking lot and didn't make it in time, and he had not had bladder control problems prior to that. We went to eat dinner at a restaurant near the dock but he couldn't sit right in the chair, was out of it, very mentally fuzzy. We had planned to watch fireworks but obviously he was not up to it, so headed back to the house and switched to the downstairs bedroom and he went to bed. He got confused getting up during the night to pee and headed out the front door before I caught him in time. He was disoriented and again didn't make it to the bathroom in time. I was getting worried now that he might have had a stroke.

July 5, 2022 – When I got up that morning, he had already been up for awhile, which is typical, and he seemed better, more alert. We talked about what had happened and he told me he had gone off cigarettes the day before, without my knowledge, and tried vaping as a substitute, and he thought he might have brought it on. So, he went out for coffee first thing and bought cigarettes, and he already felt better. We were set to do a distillery tour that morning, and he insisted he was okay to go, would take it easy. As the day went on, he seemed to get better, more like himself. Still had trouble holding his bladder at night, but otherwise was okay that day and got better every day thru the rest of the trip.

July 11,2022- Clancy called his doctor to discuss what happened on the trip, and suggests coming in for a check-up. He spoke to the nurse who says it sounds like a reaction to the vape or nicotine withdrawal "which can be powerful".

Made sense due to his improvement after resuming smoking, so we left it at that. After that, there were no incidents, but walking became more slow, balance issues too-but he took up tai chi and that helped some.

Second episode:

February 6.2023- My car broke down on the way to work and I had work commitments needing a car that day, so he picked me up and we drove back home where he called for a tow, and I took his car to work. He then took off by foot to meet the tow truck at my car, and it was cold. Apparently he lost his balance about halfway there and fell. A nice passerby saw him and stopped to help, and took him to my car to meet the tow driver, then he went home. I didn't learn about what had happened until getting home later that day. He was in some pain, so I ended up taking him to Urgent Care at KU Med, where imaging showed 4 broken ribs.

April 6, 2023- I was working in the yard. I was in the garden and had to move some rocks and I just tilted it a little bit too much and the next thing I knew I was down

on my hands and knees. But then I couldn't get up. I had 3 or 4 episodes like that. Plus it's hard to walk and Ann, my wife, bought me a cane.

Third Episode:

April 6, 2023- He was in the garden on Saturday clearing debris and bent over and lost balance and fell. I came outside and found him face down, he had no leg strength to get up. Neighbors weren't home to provide help. I struggled to help, but he was dead weight. Eventually I was able to get him onto a chair, but it took maybe 30 minutes and he was severely weakened by the effort. He called his doctor's office Monday to explain what happened and ask for neurology consult, but they scheduled him for office visit first.

April 12, 2023- Office visit with doctor, I went too and we gave full account since the Bourbon Trail episode. He set up referral w/ KU neurology. Unfortunately their earliest appt was August. Very frustrating.

Symptoms continued as weeks passed, walking turned to shuffling at some times, balance problems continued. I worry he has Parkinson's, and am getting more and more frustrated to see the neurologist, so on July 6 I call and and beg for a possible earlier appointment and snag a cancellation for that day! We go together to the appointment and the neurologist does a thorough exam, asks lots of questions but doesn't ask about family history. He says that Parkinson's is ruled out, but sees no other condition either, except blood work shows that B-12 levels are low and orders a B-12 shot and continue that each month for 4 months, and vascular imaging for legs. The B-12 shot makes a big immediate difference for his alertness and mental clarity and energy, but results are less acute for the following shots. There are no major episodes for next few months, though walking is slow and his gait is unsteady at times.

October 2023- The symptoms just kind of continue and we go on vacation, towards the fall. When we come back I was diagnosed with liver cancer with a large mass. But this whole time things were still not good. I mean, sometimes I would like lock up. This happened when we went on vacation to Kentucky, to the Bourbon Trail. And I was afraid I had a stroke.

October and November 2023-

We take a big road trip to CA in late October and though he has problems walking long stretches, we plan our activities around that and he does well on the trip. A week after returning, he starts having acute pain in his back. It comes and goes but on Monday Nov 20 he is in such pain that he goes to Urgent Care and they send him to ER for a scan. Results show a mass on his liver and thrombosis (clot) on the liver. He is admitted because of the clot, as they must use a heparin drip to keep the clot from enlarging. Saw many doctors and staff during that stay and tests were run, but no surgery or treatment on the cancer during that stay. Clancy spends Thanksgiving in the hospital and is released the day after.

November 28, 2023-We meet w/Oncologist on Tuesday. We liked him a lot. He explains that surgery is not an option so he will get Immunotherapy treatments at KU Med, one every 4 weeks. Also agreed to a clinical trial for a one time targeted radiology treatment, to break up the mass so Immunotherapy can more effectively attack the cancer.

Dec 4- Liver biopsy, outpatient, at KU Med Radiation Oncology. It goes smoothly.

Dec 12- first Immunotherapy treatment, which went well. Nurse says biopsy didn't go thru the mass, he must have another.

Dec 21- The second biopsy, had to be done on a particular machine that is in high demand which meant several hours wait. He did not bounce back after this one, movement was difficult and he was also foggy and drained. Scheduled to drive to Wisconsin for Christmas 2 days later, he was unable to make the trip, so we had to cancel. Worst Christmas ever. He continued to go downhill that week after.

December 4-21, 2023-

During the holidays we're supposed to go to Ann's sister's. I woke up the morning we were supposed to leave, and I was like, man, there's no way I can go. I was going into this clinical trial and they needed a biopsy of the tumor. And so I go in and I talk to the doctor who's going to do it. You know, some kid. I told him. I said, man, I've got a hard liver to find it's gonna be tricky, so just keep that in mind. You know, so sure enough. I get the biopsy. A couple days later, I gotta go in for treatment. The nurse tells me I have to have another biopsy. And I said, what do you mean? It's like well they got your liver, but they didn't get the mass and they need the mass for the trial.

So I go in the week before Christmas and the first one wasn't too bad, but the second one was terrible. I just

took it, dropped and total hell straight down after that one. And then it was Christmas and you know, it's the morning we're supposed to leave. And I said we're not going anywhere.

December 16,2023-Meanwhile, our niece Marsha, Ray's daughter, sent the sisters-in-laws a group text a few days later saying that Ray had fallen out of bed back home and had to get emergency services to get him off the floor. She described his condition, which was eerily similar to Clancy's recently. So I replied back to ask about the diagnosis Tim and their dad had gotten years before, since I was beginning to see a connection, after doing some online research. After reading all the replies and Doreen's vast information on NPH, it now seemed likely this was maybe Ray's and Clancy's problem too! Due to the holiday, I waited until 12/26 and tried calling the neurologist to share this info, in hopes Clancy could get an appointment right away. Tried a couple more times with no answer or call back.

January 5, 2024- We get to the first of the year 2024 and the next week, it's just pain and agony. So when Camilla, our daughter, came home on Friday, I told her to call her mother and tell her " You're gonna take me to the emergency room." And she says,"What do you need to go to the emergency room for?" I said, " I can't walk." She looks at me incredulously and says, "You can't walk? I said, " I can't walk Camilla." And then it dawned on her and she calls her mother. We go to the emergency room. They check me out and give me a CT scan. They give me a room. And then, you know, like after midnight they didn't like that CT scan, so they did an MRI.

January 2024-

So, Clancy got worse the next few days - could hardly walk, ate very little, slept a lot but couldn't even get into bed without my help, and also fell leaning over to put slippers on and I too had to call emergency services to lift him off the floor. On Jan. 5th, we took him to the ER late afternoon, as he couldn't walk. I tried telling the admitting doctors that he likely had NPH, and had to repeat the (abbreviated) history of that conclusion many times, including overwhelming family history of it. Eventually, with all the tests they ran, they did the scan that showed likelihood of NPH, and admitted him at 1 am, with an order to do a spinal tap, which is the conclusive test.

Of course, there were delays getting the lumbar puncture but the day of, which was January 6th, a therapist came and ran him thru several tests, (walking, stairs, verbal, cognitive, balance, etc.), the idea of which is to test and compare the results before and just after the procedure, the therapist came and ran him thru the tests again, and the results were staggering. She told both of us immediately that in her opinion, he definitely had NPH! He was released the next day to my surprise and was able to walk with assistance, as the puncture had relieved the extensive fluid build up. They explained that it will slowly build up again until the shunt is inserted. Now, we wait for the shunt surgery to be scheduled. It was a longer wait than I had hoped, but we finally get a call to set up a consult with his assigned neurosurgeon the following week. I accompany Clancy to the appointment, and it came with some surprises. First, the nurse sends us some signals that a shunt implant might be presumptive on our part. What?! Then the neurosurgeon comes in and tells us that Clancy's case is more complicated due to his liver cancer, since the shunt would drain to the area of his cancer. They don't know if this might cause a problem. So Clancy asks what the options are. Well, he says there is a clinical trial in the works but it might not start for a few months or more, and besides, Clancy wouldn't qualify because of the cancer. So. really no other options! And he won't "recommend" getting the shunt implant and will order it only if we insist on it, knowing there are risks. We get the message and say full steam ahead-let's get it scheduled as soon as possible.

January 6, 2024-So the next day it was just a constant parade of doctors and nurses and getting jabbed. Guy comes in and says you have this, whatever it is. Actually,

we're gonna tap your spine and so they give me a test like before and after. And the nurse that did it, she's really nice. I got the before test and then they go in and I mean this machine was just unworldly. I mean it was like science fiction, So anyway, they did it. A little bit later she comes back, gives me the test and all my everything has improved. This was all on Saturday.

They come in and they say you have NPH and we're going to put a shunt in your head. Maybe tomorrow or maybe Monday. Well it never happened. Sunday comes and they said you're getting discharged. And I go home.

So I come home after they've diagnosed me with NPH. So I have the diagnosis now. During this time, when it was really bad, I was trying to get in to see the neurologist. And I couldn't get in. They didn't answer their phones. They didn't answer their messages. I had an appointment after the first of the year already set up. So I just kept it. He really misdiagnosed me. He was the 1st Doctor at KU

that I thought was really just putting in his time, but I did get a referral. This is like the second week of January. So anyway I got the referral and he wanted to see me. We made an appointment and Ann took me and it was just as bad as you can imagine. And so when we see the guy and basically it's funny, because basically he's saying on one hand all these dire things that could happen with the procedure if things go wrong. He says we do these every week. But then on the other hand, there's some really serious consequences. I just looked at Anne and I looked at this guy and I said," You're offering me the chance to be an invalid the rest of my life. Or I could take a chance. An operation that thousands of people have every year. Come out with no problem, sir. Correctable problems. He says, yeah, that's pretty much it. I said yeah, let's do the operation. They operated and put the shunt in February 25th. So from the diagnosis which was the 7th of January to February 25th it was six weeks. That's the way they are, you just have to wait in line. When I go in for my cancer

treatment most of the time there are lots of men and women in my age range from 60 on and it's really sad. Wednesday was treatment day. There was a pre- toddler with her mother and her father. Very sad.

I got the procedure done and it was incredible. I can't even remember the next morning. I can't remember what day I got out of the hospital. I think it might have been Friday. because the next morning I got up and I looked out and saw my car. Which I hadn't driven in over a month. I said I bet I could drive. But I said maybe better give it a day. Sunday morning I got up and I said, I can definitely drive. So, I went out and drove. It was weird. I'd have to take my right hand and lift my leg up to get it over the brake pedal. I just had to be careful. From the time I got the shunt until now but especially the first months, six weeks, I mean there was improvement every single day. And it was pretty substantial at the first. By the same token, I could stand in the shower without support. Wash my hair. Wash my face. And I hadn't been able to

do that in a long time. It was great and driving, every day got better.

February 15, 2024- At long last, Clancy receives the shunt. All goes well and there are no eventual complications with the drainage, as they directed the drainage tube to the other side, away from the liver. Clancy's NPH symptoms fade with each passing week.

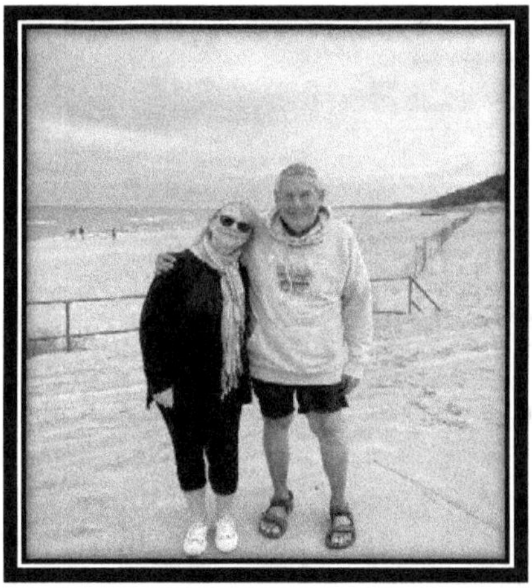

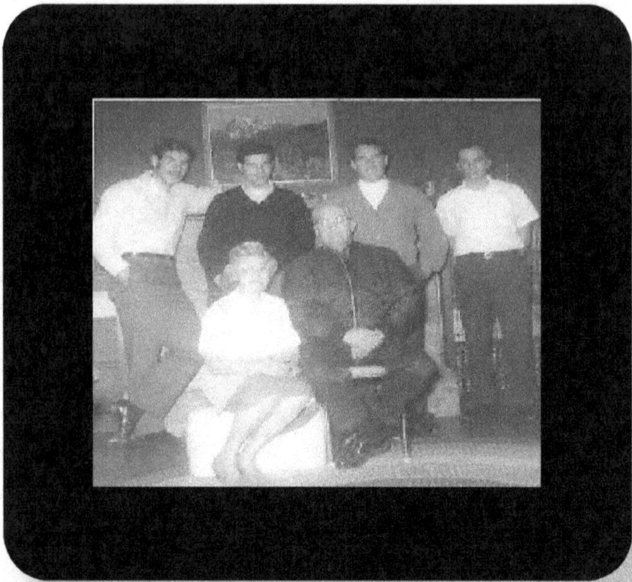

Here are all the shunt brothers after they grew up as I promised. From left to right: Tim, Pat, Casey and Ray Jr. Clancy is missing in this picture. Casey is the only one not diagnosed with NPH to this day, as well as their Mom.

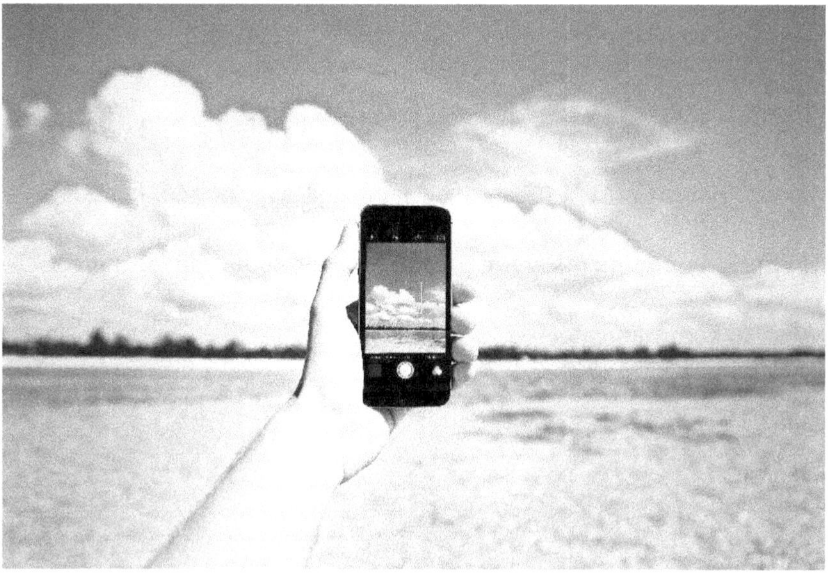

The Messenger Thread

The Wives and Daughter Tell Their Stories

8

This thread is rather long, and for that I apologize but it also has alot of great info if you are looking for a diagnosis. It is mostly about the symptoms, diagnosis, and then shunt surgery of two of the brothers. Ray had his in St. Louis at Barnes-Jewish on

Jan.27,2024 and Clancy at KU Medical Center in Kansas City on Feb.25 , 2024.

This account is told by the wives and 1 daughter: Kathy,(Pat,) Carol, (Casey), Ann, (Clancy), Marsha, (Ray) and me, Doreen (Tim). My comments are in green. Social Media can be a great way to communicate!!

Ann

This is in response to Marsha's message about Ray. Hope he is doing better. Clancy has had similar issues on occasion, lower body weakness, mentally fuzzy, etc. - and worse the last couple days. Can anyone tell me if there has been a diagnosis of this fluid on the brain that some of the brothers have? I'm seeing Hydrocephalus online and need to know if that's it. THIS IS IMPORTANT.

I need to reach out to his care team today to figure out what to do. Clancy has liver cancer- he was planning to tell the brothers last Sunday but not sure that happened. I

need to alert his care team at KU Med if he should be tested for that condition. He saw a neurologist this year but they didn't find anything, just low B-12 levels but they may have to test for it. It looks like tumors or disease made me think of this!

Sorry for long message but I need to reach out to his care team today to figure out what to do.

Thanks, Ann

Kathy

Yes, I would tell them Ann. Pat got to where he couldn't pick up his feet and couldn't remember anything. Slept a lot.

Doreen has the best information about what to look for and how to communicate with the doctors. She was a big help for me to figure it all out. If 1 doctor says he doesn't have it get another opinion.

Ann

Did Pat get the shunt Kathy? Seem to remember that he did. Thanks.

Marsha

Yes Ann, that is it. My dad was shuffling tiny baby steps but then could walk several feet with no cane. He can have a good conversation, but then can't get words for anything. Many other things as well. Dr's say it's rare and not hereditary but they'll NEVER convince me it isn't. Grandpa Cain - had a shunt, Uncle Tim - got a shunt, Pat got a shunt, my dad had a scan last year showing "mild hydrocephalus" but nothing has been done until now they're finally going to get a referral and go to Missouri for 2nd opinion/new scan.

The condition is normal pressure hydrocephalus. They will normally do a ct scan and spinal tap. Clancy did share about the liver cancer to me. So sorry he's going through this.

Good morning almost good afternoon. After Monie talked to doctor about your Dads family history. They did another CT scan. There was very little difference but said they would do a spinal tap and drain the extra fluid so they are doing that as I text. Monie is there with him and will let me know how things are when he is out from there

From Monie
Okay back in the room. Dr. Neil said normal pressure on the fluid, fluid was clear no blood. They removed a good amount of fluid and they will test it for any issues. He's resting now. Therapy is supposed to come back and walk him again. The nurse is going to get him some lunch since he didn't get to eat this morning.

RP

Hope they walked him before and after the spinal tap. That's the only way to tell of improvement. And typically they do have normal pressure thus the name"normal pressure hydrocephalus."Not playing Dr here just been thru these things.

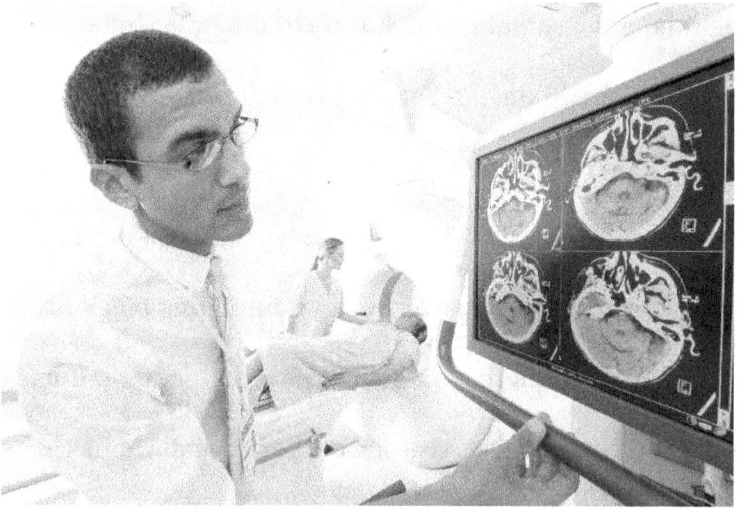

Is Clancy seeing someone at KU? Anyway I can help let me know. It's quite the ordeal.

Marsha

Like Doreen said, this is a challenging journey. When my dad had these same symptoms a year ago they finally did a CT & found the fluid but blew it off. Same symptoms this time looked at the only CT, over a year old but declined to do a new CT. ......the Dr. finally listened. They did a new CT, saw the slight change but then they went

right in, did a spinal tap and drained the fluid. It did improve his walking and clarity. A major problem is Rhonda said Illinois is at the bottom of the list for medical which I can believe. Now that this step has been done and they see improvement then we have a building block for the record. I think they're going to have to go to St. Louis and get a Neurologist. Also since Rhonda and Monie can see the difference I'd hope they're more on board with what's going on.

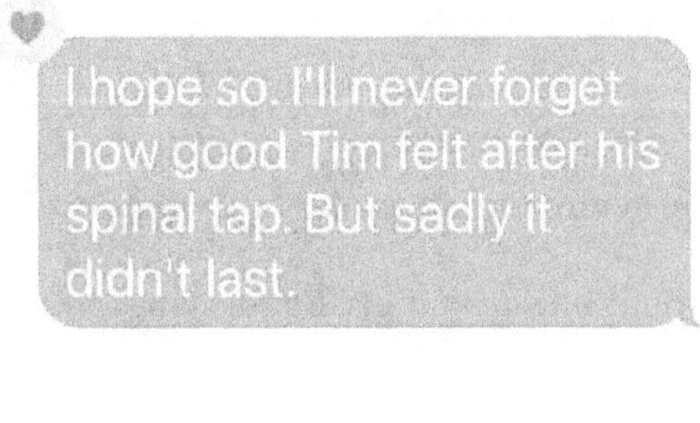

Marsha

I'm sorry you had to do all the research and take the lead but THANK YOU!!!

I'm just sorry for all the years Tim went thru this and I was pretty sure what was wrong but nobody listened. The research was nothing but THANK YOU for all your help to both of us over the yrs!

Ann

It sounds like this diagnosis must happen thru a neurologist, so I hope Ray can get a referral soon. Clancy already has a neurologist- now we're just waiting for a call back from him so they can get him in and confirm the NPH. I appreciate all your input, especially Doreen, as that info will be helpful when we have the appointment. Prayers to all going thru health issues.

> That's the way they want you to do it but we went to 7 neurologists and none of them diagnosed it. And forget VA. A neurosurgeon agreed to see Tim and agreed he had excess fluid and might benefit from a shunt. Then we went to Mayo Clinic and they confirmed the diagnosis. Hope you get a good neurologist. I think Pat got his diagnosis from a primary care Dr who sent him to a neurosurgeon if I remember right. Yes prayers appreciated!

You went to see seven neurologists Doreen? Do you know why they resist that particular diagnosis? That is disturbing! We liked the neurologist at Landon Center but we will see what he says about this. I'm concerned now that this diagnosis may be difficult to get.

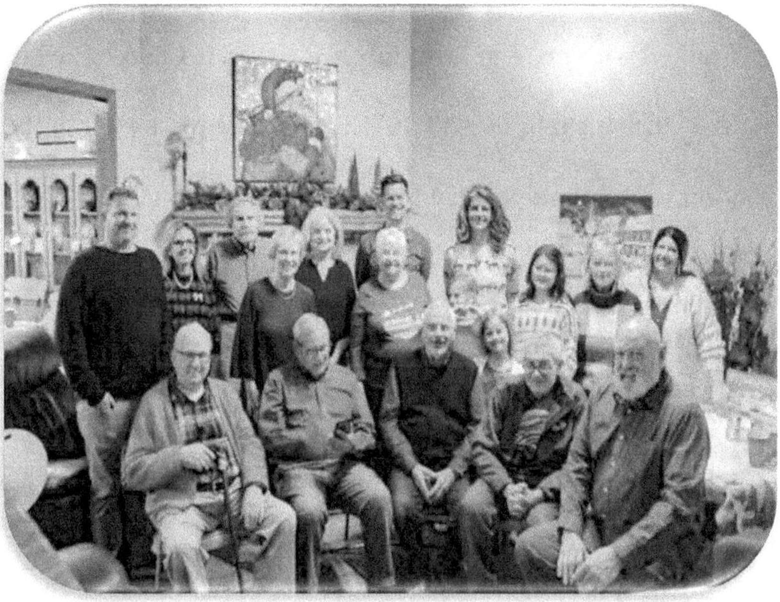

The Family Christmas December 2023. Two brothers would be diagnosed with NPH in early 2024. The brothers in front row L/R: Ray, Casey, Pat, Clancy and Tim (in back with gray shirt). And the wives and daughter in this thread: L/R: Marsha (Ray), Carol (Casey), Doreen (Tim), Kathy (Pat) and Ann (Clancy) second from right.

Marsha

I talked with my dad last night. He asked if I had talked to him since his fall. WHAT FALL? Apparently he fell in the kitchen at home. I asked about it but he said he was having trouble with his words. I messaged Rhonda. I let him know three firemen passed away. Two were close friends for many years. All of a sudden he was hyped up telling me a story about one of them with details!! I'm perplexed.

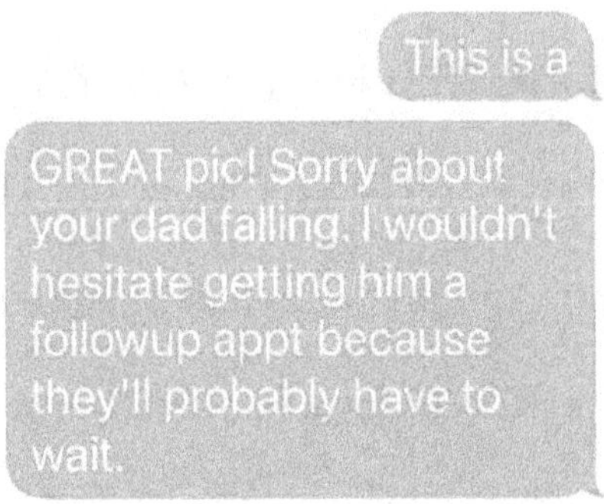

Ann

I've been trying to get an appointment since 12-26 to discuss the family history and he is clearly showing those symptoms, so hopefully he will test Clancy for it and order the shunt. Clancy could barely walk tonight.

Kathy

When it rains it pours. Will pray that everything goes well when he gets his shunt. It has really made a big difference in Pat. Take care of yourself too.

Ann

Yeah, I guess it does. The NPH and the cancer together is a tough combo. I sure wish we would have realized the NPH was what he had when we first saw the neurologist in July. He would have more strength to

fight the cancer now if he had the shunt. Thanks, will sure take those prayers, too.

Ann

In the ER tonite, brought him here about 5 pm. Clancy was so weak he couldn't walk at all. He fell early this morning when he got out of bed and bent over to get his shoes on and lost balance. Had to call EMTs to get him off the floor (just like Ray), and guess it took any strength he had out of him. They did a CT scan and said if he has NPH it should show up, but I'm dubious from what Doreen has said. We will see. They will likely admit him but unless they see the NPH, not sure how long they would keep him for balance and weakness.

Carol

I'm so sorry about all of this. Let us know if we can help. We're going to Springfield tomorrow, but will be back sometime Sunday. If he needs rides to appointments, let us know or if you need an extra person to go with you to the doctor, we can help. Prayers for Clancy and you. I hope you can get some answers soon.

Kathy

Oh this is sad news. Pat's doctor diagnosed him, but didn't rely on just a ct scan. You may want to insist that they do the other tests while he is in there.

Ann

They admitted him about 1 am this morning, after 8 hrs in the ER. He's having lumbar puncture sometime today, already had an MRI this morning. They explained how it will work just as you described Doreen, (thank you for that) I left hospital at 2:30 this morning and heading back

there soon. Pray for the results we need from the puncture and getting a shunt soon!

The CT Scan was what led them to the possibility of NPH, that's why they admitted him. The Neurologist on-call wasn't 100% on it tho and took his time to make that decision! They have delayed the puncture until Monday now, to make sure the blood thinner is out of his system. Just hope and pray it shows the results we need and that he gets a shunt! Thanks for all your care, help and support.

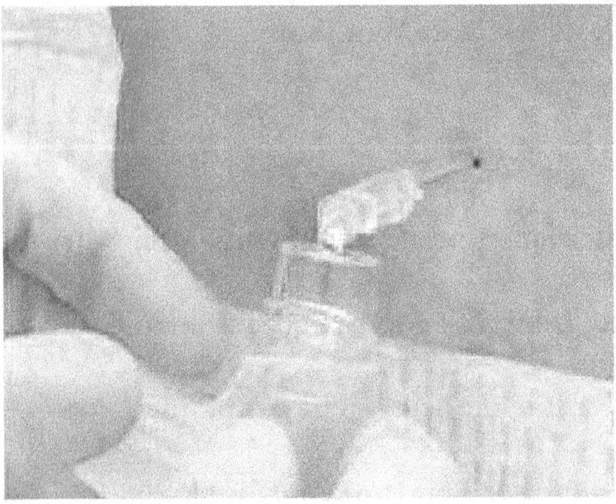

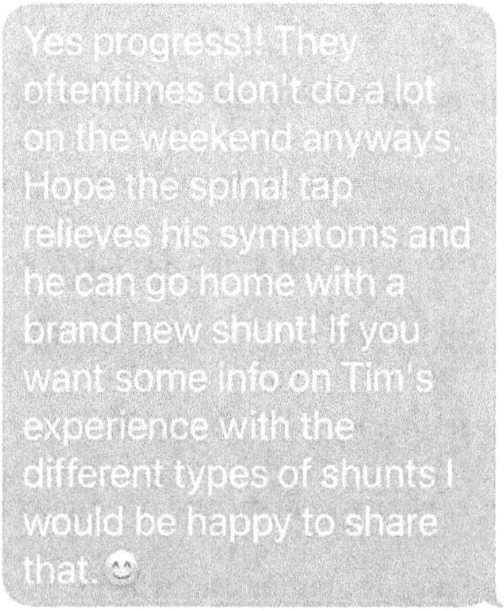
Yes progress!! They oftentimes don't do a lot on the weekend anyways. Hope the spinal tap relieves his symptoms and he can go home with a brand new shunt! If you want some info on Tim's experience with the different types of shunts I would be happy to share that. 😊

Marsha

How does one know when it's right and to push for a shunt? I know we need to somehow get him a neurologist for starts. I don't know if that might be St. Louis or Kansas City.

Ann

It was quite a process to get here, ironically the unexpected ER visit Friday ended up being a good thing. We first had to go to his primary care who agreed to make a referral to a neurologist- but it took MONTHS to get an appointment! Meanwhile Clancy was getting worse. I finally in desperation called to see if anything earlier was open and got an actual person who had just had a cancellation. But when we saw the neurologist we didn't make the family history connection and we weren't asked if there was family history. So he just ruled out a couple things, and didn't bring up NPH as a possibility. It's a tough diagnosis to get because it generally comes after age 70 and the symptoms get passed off as dementia, as we know. But he has to go through a neurologist to be diagnosed, which Ray should be able to get if he's on Medicare.

Ann

Just know that the population is aging and there is a long wait (at least here) to get those appointments- Very frustrating.

Marsha

Thank you for the info and sharing your journey as well. I'm sorry you're going through all of this. Just like Tim has been so blessed to have Doreen to be a voice for him and amazing research skills, I'm glad Clancy has you doing all you are for him. Yes, I did read they generally are diagnosed after age 70. It boggles my mind that it's pretty "uncommon" yet we have 5 out of 6 immediate relatives with it. Yes! I find myself questioning is this "Age / Alzheimer's / Dementia" vs NPH but the Cat Scan showed a mild amount over a year ago. When they changed lanes and decided to go ahead with new scan they did see "change" & while it sounded like it was being minimized the very next morning he was having a spinal

tap and fluid drained. He has all 3 symptoms and because it's not consistent I feel like I should move this forward. Being almost 84 is concerning for surgery but we don't want permanent brain damage either from not draining it. It just occurred to me that at the Christmas gathering Tim was trying to tell me the pecan pie I took him was really good. He said he was having trouble with his words but I picked up on what he was saying and we figured it out. The other evening my dad said almost the exact same thing. Having trouble with his words but he was trying to tell me about his fall.

Ann

Yes, to all you said Marsha! To me, the key symptom is the "shuffling feet" and lower body weakness. And slow speech and cognitive difficulties. Clancy is the youngest of

the brothers yet these symptoms became progressively worse in the last couple months, probably due to tumor.

Ann

Update: Clancy had lumbar puncture this morning! It wasn't painful and the tests before and after indicated NPH and that a shunt is recommended! However, we haven't heard where or when. I'm hoping they can do it while he's here- neurosurgery resident who stopped in told Clancy they can implant them on an outpatient basis. But this was a very big day!

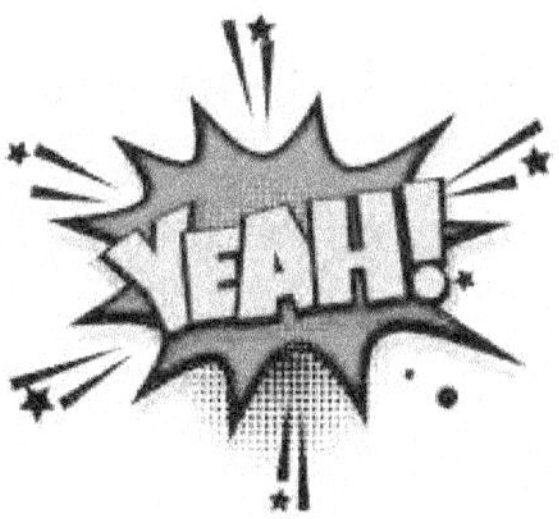

Kathy

Great that they got him diagnosed. When Pat had his he had to stay in ICU for 3 days. Guess they have improved how they put them in.

Marsha

What tests has he had done today besides Lumbar Puncture. Same as spinal tap? He said he's fallen 2-3 times recently "and HARD" Rhonda is there and corrected him it's been once. I let him know about Clancy and started the conversation that we need to see a neurologist and he might need to get one. I'm glad Clancy

is getting what he needs.

Carol

It was a big day! Hard to believe 3 brothers and maybe 4, with Ray, all have this condition. I'm sure all the information you had helped to move things more quickly.

Marsha- The MRI confirmed the enlarged ventricles, which then led to them ordering the lumbar puncture (LP), where they drain off most of the excess fluid. The physical therapist ran him thru several tests (timed walking, memory, cognitive, etc) before the LP, and then repeated the exact tests after the LP, which measured if there were measurable differences in the before and after. That shows if NPH is causing the problems.

Good morning your Dad had his appointment with new neurologist in MO yesterday. The doctor in the hospital got on the ball and he and the primary got your Dad pushed through the schedule quickly. This neuro actually started his career in studies of this particular condition. Monie really liked him.
He has one more pre-op appointment and then the surgery will be scheduled at Barnes hospital sometime this month. No date. The doctor felt like your Dad met all the criteria for having it and 90% of people profit by it. I have no more information and I have no date yet but will let you know as soon as we get one. Would you be able to be here for the procedure? It will be an overnight stay.

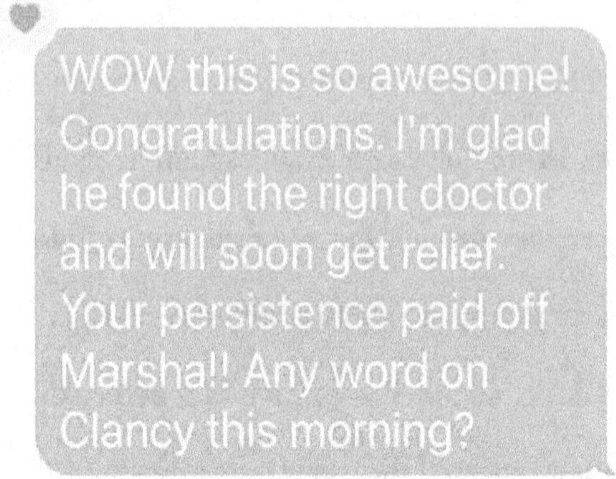

Marsha

WELLLLLLL, sure would be nice to have KNOWN this but WOOHOO THEY'RE FINALLY LISTENING, and the ball is rolling in high speed ..... check this message out that I just received!!!!

Ann

Wow!! This is great news Marsha! Can't believe he got in to a neurologist so fast and that is unbelievable that he got one who is knowledgeable on NPH! Keep

me posted on the type of shunt. Did they do the lumbar puncture? We are still waiting on getting the shunt scheduled but Clancy is moving around and drove himself to a doctor's appt this morning, and will have another one this afternoon.

Marsha

Yes, they did. I've BEEN saying I believe these symptoms are not just Covid. I believe he needs rechecked & a Neurologist. This recent hospital stay we were going to have to go to the primary, get a referral, go through the red tape but then things changed instantly. They changed their mind and did the cat scan, basic testing, the next morning he was having the lumbar puncture, fluid drained and a week later here we are.

Carol

This family probably should have a case study done. I think it's very unusual for 4 out of 5 (and who knows about number 5) siblings to be diagnosed with NPH.

Marsha

Exactly!! I've thought that as well. And with Grandpa having it as well. 5 out of 6 immediate relatives.

Ann

Carol, I feel the same way! This has to be an oddity and would seem to some value in the research of this condition! Marsha, that's a good point. Since they are an all male sibling group, you have to wonder.

There was a resident from KU we saw at VA who was very interested in doing research on this and asked if he could access Tim's medical records. I said he could use whatever he wanted and that's the last I heard from him. But when they say it's not hereditary they are wrong!

Ann

Yes, and what I found during our ordeal in the ER and hospital is that no one paid much attention when I informed them of the family history!

Marsha

Doreen, from the moment that Dr. said there's no way this is hereditary I said it then and to this day I will NEVER be convinced that it isn't. Also, it looks like they're changing their tune toward this but it feels like this could be a record to be studied.

Ann

Clancy is meeting with his "regular" neurologist today and I'm going to be sure he mentions this. He is the one who missed the NPH in July and this is just a regular follow up appt, nothing to do with the recent happenings. But he is also with KU Med.

Marsha

Ann, we've learned from Tim's many trips, Dr.'s, tests and experiences that an NPH patient needs a

cheering squad speaking up for them. I'm glad I've been able to "get through" and be heard even from afar. Doreen, I don't know where we would all be if you had not done the research and spoke up to the doctors.

Carol

Doreen, I agree. You have given everybody a real heads up on this condition.

Marsha

Exactly!! It would be so interesting to know how many doctors you have helped educate while saving yourself and Tim. It seemed there was always an excuse, brush it aside, overlook and just not listen / try on their part but you made many things happen for the good.

Marsha

I hope Clancy's appointments went well today. Too bad he and my dad couldn't get their shunts together. Family discount? I know there's nothing funny about this just looking for a lighter side. never know........ could happen.

Well they were diagnosed within days of each other so will have a lot in common.

Marsha

I truly believe they should do a case study. I asked for my dad's new Neurosurgeon" s name and waiting for that. It's a long way but I would like to go to his appointment and I informed Rhonda that weather permitting I plan to be there for his surgery at Barnes Jewish. Since he is very familiar with NPH I'm confident he can answer some questions and perhaps direct us for a case study.

Marsha

I would like help to create a list of questions for this new Dr. who is so familiar with NPH. What should I ask?

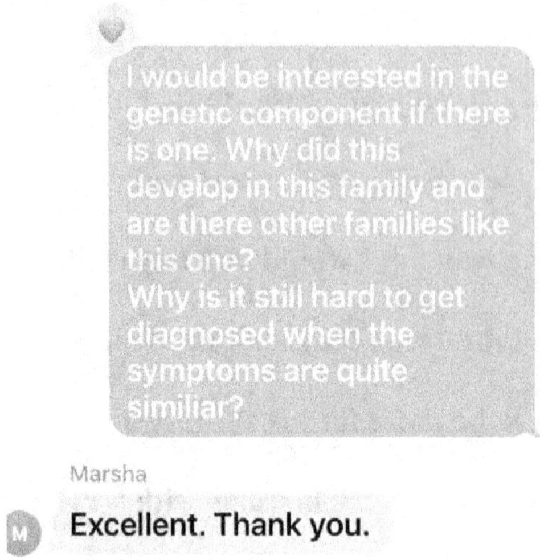

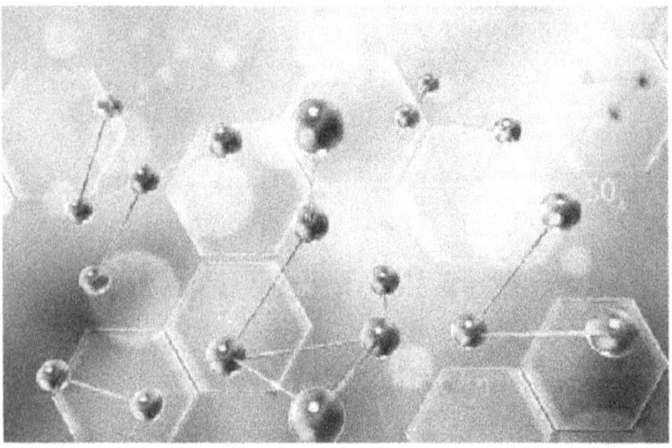

Ann

So glad to hear that Marsha!! We still haven't seen anything about getting Clancy's scheduled.

Ann

Btw, Clancy went yesterday for his second Immunotherapy treatment and we met with his oncologist and talked about the NPH diagnosis. He said he would make a call to help get the shunt going, since it still had not been scheduled over a week later! When we got home the Neurosurgery dept called to give us a surgery date!

Sadly, the soonest date is Feb 27th. So, we are on the waiting list for possible cancellations. That is a long time to wait as he needs every bit of strength he can get to fight this cancer. Pray for a cancellation soon please.

Carol **Ann, we were just thinking about Clancy and how things were progressing. We'll pray for a cancellation soon.**

Marsha

All appointments cancelled today at both locations. 1 set is rescheduled for tomorrow and working on the others. Trimming strings from his pants this morning, lost his balance, slow motion sideways then fell. I broke the fall and from hitting his head on the stove/counter but was a few steps too far to be more help. He is to use his walker at all times now. A few hallucinations / seeing things.

Ann

Clancy meets with the neurosurgeon tomorrow and if he doesn't get this shunt scheduled soon, Clancy said they will be seeing him in the ER again soon! The struggle is real.

Marsha

Ann, how did Clancy's appointment go?

Ann

It went well. He is going to coordinate with the Oncology team to schedule the shunt at the best time for optimal immunity, based on Clancy's schedule for his cancer treatments. He wanted to inform us of the possible risks considering Clancy's cancer. As he told us, a shunt surgery is common and for an otherwise healthy person, fairly simple. For Clancy, there are some risks involved. I said I hoped the consultation with the cancer team would happen as quickly as possible!! How is your dad doing today?

Marsha

Today was overall good. Asked questions to the Dr.

* No idea of gender, genetic, environment or other correlation.

* No need to change shunts until there are symptoms regardless of how long it's been in.

* No there are not any known tests ahead of time.

* No he's not aware of a case study however he has NEVER EVER seen anything like our family.

He's an excellent Dr. but there are so many unknowns.

Going over the small 1% - 5% chance of various things happening has my dad a little worked up. He feels like it's a huge thing and if he had known this he'd never have signed up. I told him that hopefully after the procedure and he starts noticing a difference (4 - 6 weeks) then he'll be glad he did it.

Good morning, I want to thank you all for sharing and caring amongst us. I appreciate having this chat

thread as it's basically my only connection, encouragement etc. It's been a challenge getting the shunt concern / info to the Dr but he will get my message between surgery today! We'll see what he says. We have several pre- op things today at Barnes Jewish.

My dad said maybe the family can all get together for all the brothers and their shunts. I think he means at least spring time.

Ann

Marsha, it will be so helpful for Clancy and I hearing the reports on your dad's surgery, considering how close it is to Clancy's! One thing we learned yesterday which Doreen probably knows is that the shunt procedure was used primarily for pediatric cases, and kids have fewer risks. The surgery itself hasn't changed much over time, and does have

complications for older people - which sounds like your dad wasn't expecting- so there are risks. In Clancy's case, even more risks specific to his type of cancer. There is a less invasive treatment that is fairly close to being approved (they are doing clinical trials now) but the timeline is still not soon enough to be an option for us! Don't know if that was mentioned by your dad's doctor. Keep us posted! Will be praying for good outcome tomorrow and in the days/weeks ahead!

Had to get a wheelchair today.

EKG shows he is in Afib.

Marsha

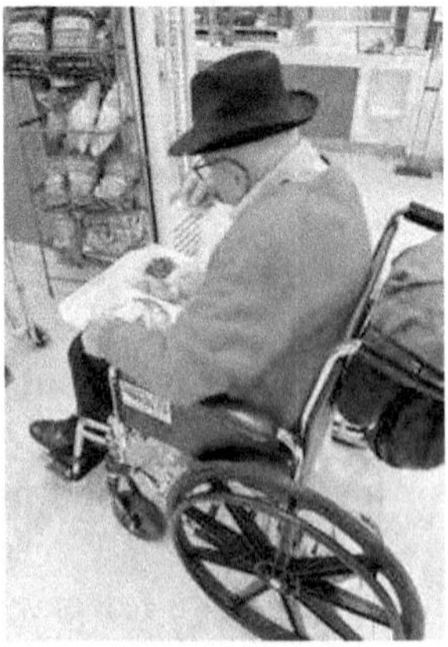

Delay Delay Delay......

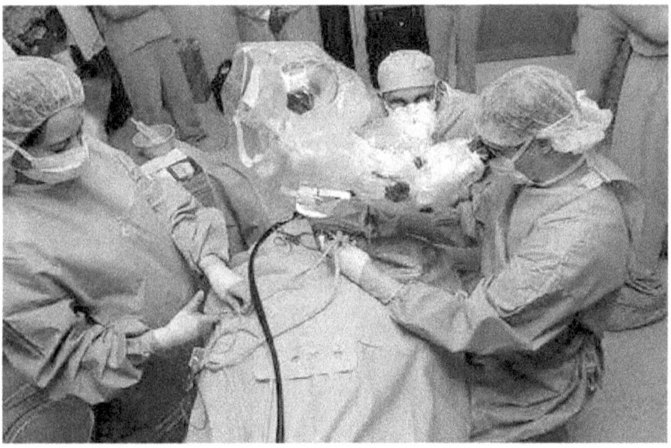

GOOOO time

They JUST took him back.

Surgery is done.

Said he did great! No problems, he's getting woken up now, I'll see him in recovery in about 45 min.

(Doreen, his setting is at 1.5 & they'll monitor from there) They have CT's & X-ray's for a baseline and placement. Inner sutures with outer staples. All is good at the moment. No ICU needed which was not known earlier.

Kathy

Good to hear that everything went well. Are they keeping him just overnight? Pat's is set at 4. He did have to go to ICU. Because they had to drain so much fluid before they put the shunt in. Will he get to go back to his house?

Marsha

Yes he'll be here overnight. Dr. anticipates he'll be released tomorrow but we have to wait and see. Make sure he's eating, feeling ok, etc. They just drained his fluid and don't want to drain it too fast.

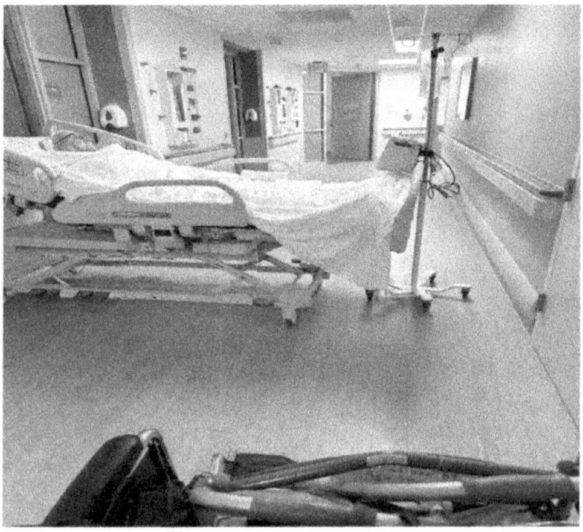

THANK YOU!! I'm getting his favorite sausage gravy biscuit breakfast, then heading home!!

Is it typical for fluctuation in thinking. During the day, waiting for surgery, it was getting harder for him to think, answer questions and speak. After surgery and getting checked into his room he was sharp and firm in his answers. Now, he doesn't know he had surgery, until he's told or "shunt" is mentioned. Says it hurts but doesn't want to complain & he'll be alright. As soon as I gave him medication he asked if he was going to get something for it. Etc. I called last evening & said I was checking

on him. He asked if I thought he had been sick. It feels like we jumped into full fledged Alzheimer's. Yes, the Dr. said 4-6 weeks. This is considerably worse than 1 week ago though. I didn't know if it might dip down then back up or what is going on. When looking rhrough the MyChart apparently he has had concern for years and did have some testing done but I'm still sorting through things. I just thought I'd put it out there and ask.

Kathy

Pat did that too but it got better real quick. He is acting like that now that's why I think he needs an adjustment.

Ann **Good news here- Clancy is scheduled for shunt surgery on Feb 15th! That was their soonest available and that date will allow him to get his radiation**

treatment, 3rd immunotherapy treatment and his appointment with vascular doctor in beforehand.

Hope Ray is continuing to improve.

Marsha

Graphic pic warning – just sharing healing in 12 days

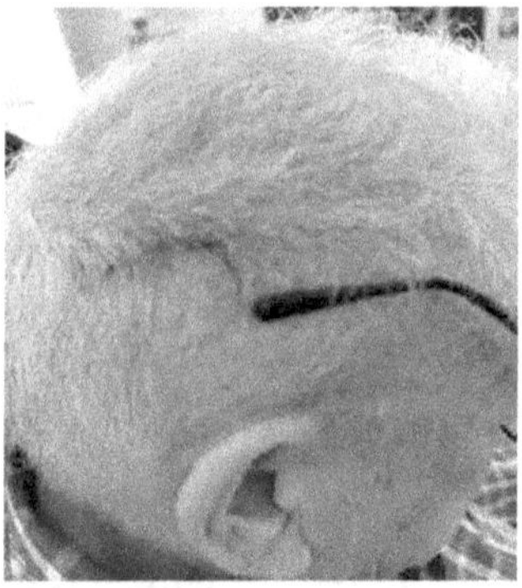

2/14/2024 6:05:36

Marsha

Ann, would you let Clancy know I'm thinking of him and saying a prayer for his surgery. He'll do great.

Ann

Thank you Marsha! Will keep everyone posted how it goes tomorrow.

Ann

He is in surgery now. Was finally able to ask the Neurosurgeon right before what kind of shunt he was getting. He looked at me funny and asked "do you mean which brand?" It's a Codman programmable. The surgery resident was kinda amazed to hear Clancy is the fourth of his brothers to get one. The surgeon doesn't understand I have a whole "consulting team" where types of shunts have been discussed at length!

Marsha **YouGO girl!**

Yes 4 of 5 brothers but also it started with their father so they are 2nd generation.

Ann

Yep, mentioned that too! We can all compare shunt stories at next Cain gathering! Crazy.

Marsha

How are things going?

Ann

Very well! He is walking better already. I expect to see steady progress, not a big jump- because the drainage will be at level 5 to see how that goes. He got a CT scan and X-ray this afternoon and hope for good results so he will be released tomorrow! Marsha, your dad called. Carol and Casey were here so we all talked to him. He sounds like things are good!

AWES

Yes that sounds really good! We are very happy for him!

2/15/2024 8:24:51

Kathy

This is good news. You will see improvement, but will take a couple of weeks to be normal. Glad he finally got his.

Marsha

ME TOO!! 5 out of 6 - so far is CRAZINESS. Glad to hear he's doing better!

Kathy

Pat had the headaches and dizziness right after he got his. Went back to the surgeon and he just adjusted the shunt. It's so nice when they get better from the initial surgery. Men are not usually the best at being a patient. This time next year we will all be on the downhill side. Yeah!

Ann

Yes, when I did my initial research I read about familial NPH, which I figured was newer (since your experience with Tim), but they still don't seem to make a strong case for it!

I would be surprised if there WASN'T headache, honestly but it isn't that bad, he just takes Tylenol. He has a follow up appointment on the calendar with the(neurosurgeon) and if he still has them then, maybe that's a consideration.

How are all the shunt brothers doing this week? And how is Tim doing from the knee surgery Doreen?

Clancy had an appt with neurosurgeon nurse to check his wound and all is going well! He still has some headache and she said- "well, they did drill a hole in your head" so I guess that means a little headache for a while is expected. He meets with the neurosurgeon in 2 weeks I think and then we should know whether an adjustment is needed.

Marsha

"I spoke to the Dr.'s nurse about my dad's headaches and the new change after the shunt adjustment. It was in the right temple. I was told it was normal but if Tylenol stopped working then it was a problem. WELLLL.... My dad just heard back about his cat scan and they want him in the office NOW for a shunt adjustment. My guess is over shunting but why would it takes this long for results when the Dr. already saw it to verify setting and placement. I hope for the best.

Marsha

Ok! I just called St. Louis and spoke with a nurse. The "fluid" is actually a small brain bleed. He's adjusted back to 1.5 & will repeat the cat scan in 2 weeks. The something line is stable and has not shifted so it's not moving any brain tissue. Because of you, Doreen, I can feel a little more on top of things. talking with the nurse & Dr. Thank you for all you've shared in this journey. It's been a tremendous help for me to help my dad.

Good morning everyone. I have some exciting news. Well for me anyways. I am writing a book! The title is "The Shunt Brothers: A story of familial NPH. I have been researching for awhile and it is in the works.
It is mostly a family story and this is where I need some help:
1. I need some personal stories of what you went thru prior to the shunt. I am not including Drs names but will talk about hospitals. I am quoting Drs notes verbatim from Tim's records. Highlighted the misdiagnosis for yrs.
2. I need permission to use first names and pics of the family. If you have any to share that would be great.

Ann

Amazing that you are doing this, Doreen! No one better to do it, and with Brandon's help you will have the guidance that you DIDN'T have on the shunt journey! And it will give the next generation all that family health history, which is important.
I will talk to Clancy about it tonight. Proud of you for doing this!

Carol

Great idea, Doreen. Casey will write what he remembers about his dad. He also wants to pre-order your book when it's ready.

Marsha

me toooo! I'd love you to autograph it as well.

Kathy

KC This sounds like a good project. Will pass the information on to Pat.

Marsha

Awesome!!! Congratulations & THANK YOU. Absolutely I will send you info, pics, etc. I love the title They'll always be "The Shunt Brothers" to me!

Part Two

Learning About CT Scans and Shunts

and Other Symptoms

Learning About CT Scans

9

I would like to delve into the importance of knowing a little bit about CT scans and their appearance when there is Normal Pressure Hydrocephalus. I would never speak up to a doctor when the inevitable report came back reading "no hydrocephalus". I just accepted it as fact and that's as far as it would go. I never once talked to a radiologist or questioned their reading of the CT scan. I realized I had no training and wouldn't recognize it on the scans anyway. I very seldom even was shown Tim's CT scan images, just the report. So then I got a little more educated and with a lot of research I began to question these findings. There is plenty of information about the appearance of NPH on CT scans available on the internet. I would get the images, load them up on a computer, take a few screenshots and compare them. I realize no professional likes to be questioned about his findings, so I had to tread lightly so to speak.

I began putting the CT screenshots into a large 3 ring binder and labeling dates and any other info that I thought might be helpful. I got some strange looks when I took it in for doctor's visits, but at this point I really didn't care. It was better to have something concrete to show them than an elusive image on a computer and many of these were from years ago.

In order to have a comparison to normal size ventricles, I offer some scans of my own MRI. I was not suffering from NPH but I did have some concerning vision loss. Then I will share Tim's MRI and CT Scans and compare them to his brother's scans who were suffering from symptoms and these were their last images before their diagnosis.

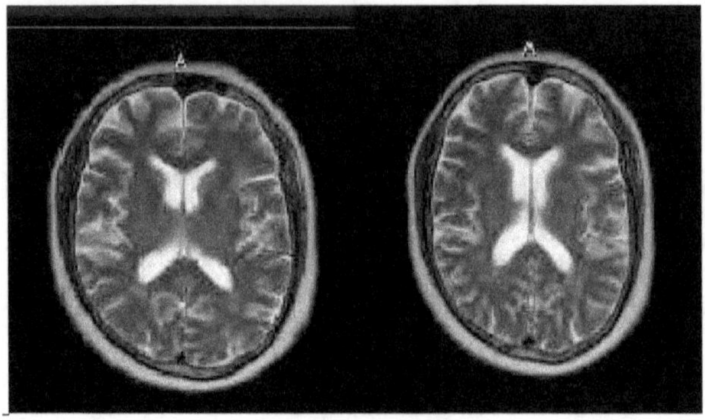

Figure 1: Doreen's Normal MRI 01/08/2019

Some of Tim's images go way back to 2008 with an MRI. It's hard to believe he had NPH for all these years, but it looks like this was the case. Then we jump to 2010 which also was misdiagnosed. Then 2012 which was also misdiagnosed. Notice a pattern here?

Tim's final imaging was in 2014 the year he was correctly diagnosed with NPH at Mayo Clinic. So there were quite a few neurologists and other doctors who looked at these images. Absolutely astounding that not one of them interpreted NPH. I guess they can claim it was "unknown" but that claim is a little ridiculous to me.

It is rather easy to see the difference in the CT scans. I don't think you need to be a radiologist to recognize the size difference. The ventricles most affected are the lateral ventricles, and the third and fourth ventricles.

Figure 2: Tim's MRI 4/17/2008

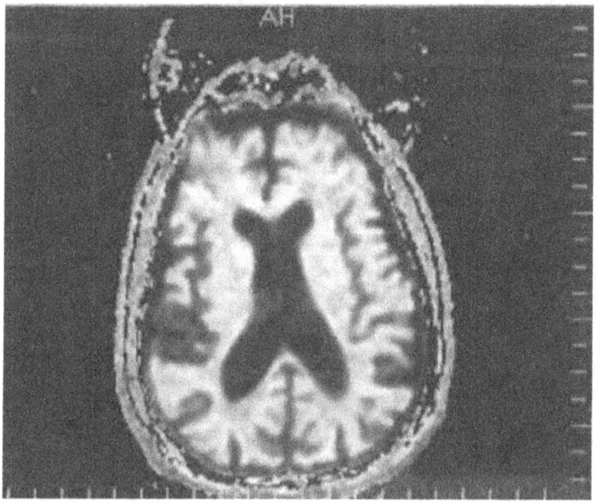

Tim's Radiology Report : 4/17/08

```
Findings: The ventricles and sulci are
unremarkable. No
effacement of sulci is noted. There is no
evidence of acute
hemorrhage, infarction or midline shift. No
abnormal patterns of
contrast enhancement detected. A few
scattered periventricular
white matter lesions are seen bilaterally
consistent with small
vessel ischemic changes.
```

Figure 3: Clancy's MRI 1/5/2024

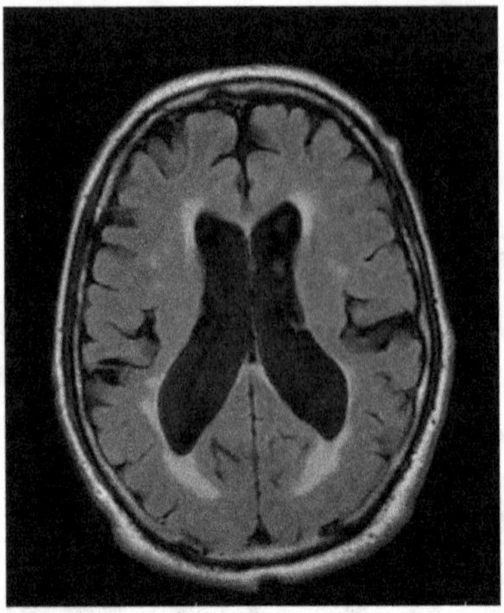

Clancy's Radiology Report: 1/5/24

HISTORY: WEAKNESS.FALL

Impression

1. **No acute intracranial abnormality.**

2. **Redemonstration of disproportionate lateral ventricular enlargement with sulcal crowding at the vertex and acute callosal angle which may be seen in normal pressure hydrocephalus in the appropriate clinical setting.**

3. **Mild nonspecific white matter disease, likely due to chronic microvascular ischemia.**

To my untrained eye these scans look almost alike, but Tim's looks like he has more fluid buildup. And Tim had to wait six more long years for a diagnosis, while Clancy was diagnosed the next day. Improvements in diagnosis? Maybe but the misdiagnosis numbers are still dismal.

Figure 4: Tim's CT Scan: 6/18/2010

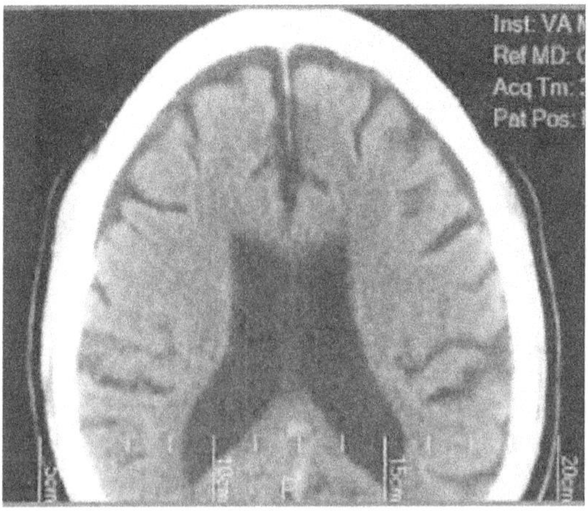

Tim's Radiology Report: 6/18/2010

Findings: There is mild cortical atrophy with prominence of ventricles and sulci. No effacement of the sulci is seen. There is no evidence of acute hemorrhage, infarction or midline shift. No extra-axial fluid collections are present.

Visualized bony structures are intact.

Figure 5: Ray's CT Scan: 12/21/2023

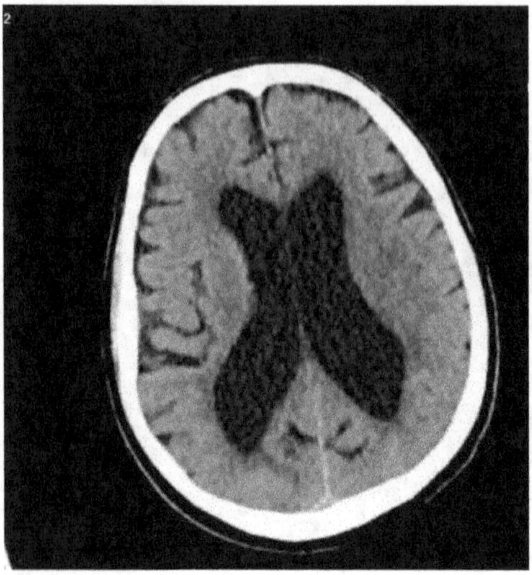

Ray's Radiology Report:12/21/2023

Impression:

No acute intracranial findings.

Crowding of the sulci at the vertex and prominence to mild enlargement of the ventricles appears unchanged since 2022. Findings can sometimes be seen in the setting of normal pressure hydrocephalus.

Tim had another four years to suffer symptoms and Ray got his surgery and a shunt in less than a month in January of 2024. An astute observer might ask why he was not diagnosed in 2022 if the ventricles appeared the same. That will be answered a little later in the book titled: "Anatomy of a misdiagnosis." To wrap this all up, in ensuing years, Tim had symptoms leading to a CT scan and then puzzled doctors offered no diagnosis or the wrong diagnosis. The last two are from 2012 and 2014 with excerpts from his radiology reports.

Figure 6:Tim's CT Scan 12/03/2012

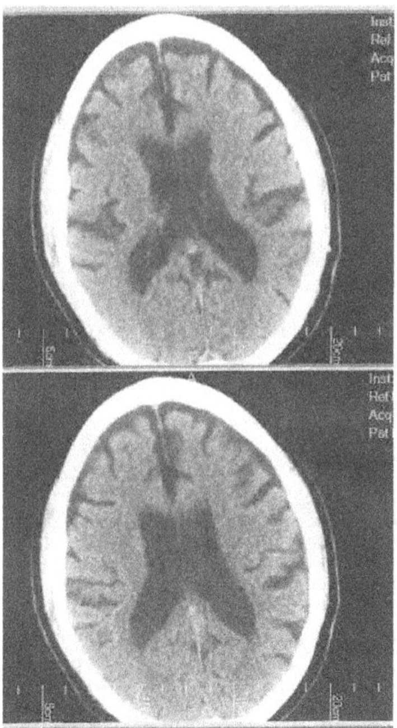

Tim's Radiology Report: 12/03/2012

```
Clinical History: altered mental status

Comparison: Head CT 06/18/2010

Findings: No intracranial hemorrhage,
hydrocephalus or brain
herniation.
```

Figure 7: Tim's CT Scan 5/30/2014

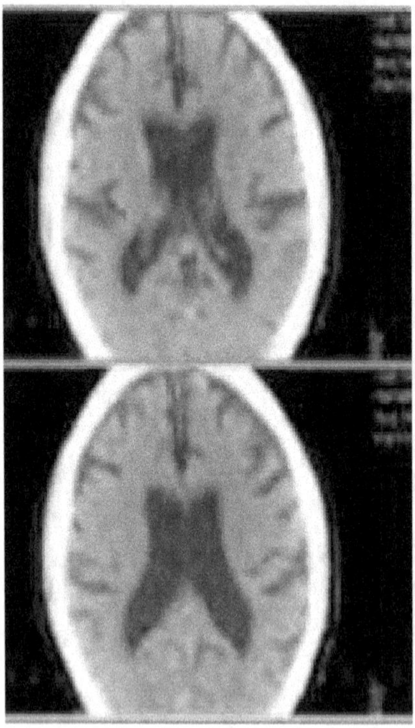

Tim's Radiology Report: 5/30/2014

```
Findings:  Moderate diffuse brain atrophy is
noted with prominent
extra-axial spaces bases. Ventricular megaly
is in proportion the
amount of brain atrophy. Mild to moderate
chronic white matter
ischemic changes also.
```

It seems their favorite go-to excuse for the ventriculomegaly is brain atrophy or central brain atrophy. That explains everything doesn't it?

Figure 8: Tim's CT Scan 8/17/15 After Shunt Placement

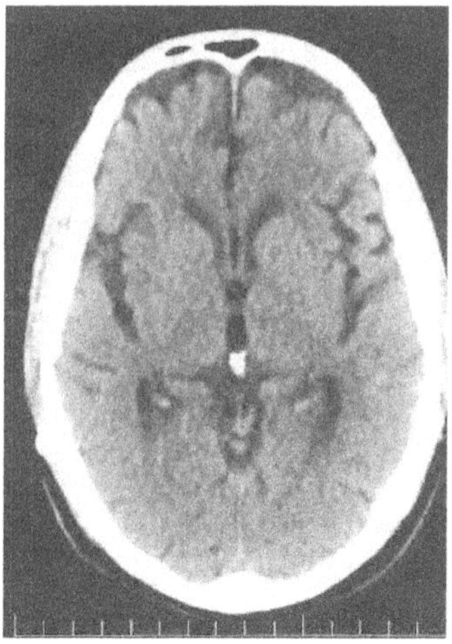

So it seems pretty obvious that Tim had excess fluid in the ventricles dating back to 2008.

That would be 6 years before he was diagnosed and got his first shunt. Wow, it seems like this is pretty close to a major medical mistake. The only one who suffered however was my husband. I only regret I had no knowledge of what was going on and didn't ask enough questions.

Some notable comments from the radiology reports dating back to the MRI in 2008.

2008- Clinical History: Dizziness, Loss of Equilibrium, Sluggish

"The ventricles and sulci are unremarkable" Translation: Totally normal, nothing to see here. No explanation for your symptoms.

2010- Clinical History: Headache and memory" impairment

"There is mild cortical atrophy with prominence of ventricles and sulci" Translation: The ventricles and sulci are enlarged but we have no idea why and this is as far as our expertise goes. No worries.

2012-

Clinical History: altered mental status

- Findings: "No intercranial hemorrhage. Hydrocephalus or brain herniation" Translation: Yes, the ventricles are still enlarged, but no worries. Nothing to see here, move along. That is if you can pick up your feet. Sorry about that shuffling walk and pain. We don't have any idea what's causing it.

Keep in mind Tim was 60 – 64 years old when he was having these difficulties. I've read that NPH is most common in the elderly, especially those in their 80s. He was 20 years younger than this with debilitating symptoms. So there are probably plenty of younger patients who could be helped with the right diagnosis.

2014-

- Findings: " Moderate diffuse brain atrophy is noted with prominent diffuse extra-axial spaces bases. Ventriculomegaly is in proportion to the amount of brain atrophy. So after all these years of repeated ct scans and all these years of debilitating symptoms, there was really no explanation for his worsening symptoms.

Undiagnosed NPH can cause damage to the frontal lobe. It appears that this is what happened to my husband for all these years. It was barely mentioned when discussing his symptoms and CT results. This is the brain region most significantly affected by the excess cerebrospinal fluid buildup, leading to cognitive impairments like difficulty with decision making, planning, and behavioral changes if left untreated. Essentially the pressure from the excess fluid can damage the frontal lobe responsible for these functions.

The frontal lobe is considered the primary area affected by NPH. It leads to prominent symptoms like apathy, impaired executive function, and changes in personality. If left undiagnosed, the frontal lobe damage can worsen over time.

Well we had plenty of time for the excess fluid to do its damage, as Tim was undiagnosed for many years. I will delve more into personality and behavior changes in the next section, but he certainly was affected and exhibited all of the problems that frontal lobe damage can do to the brain. Very sad and also infuriating to the caretaker who doesn't understand what is taking place. Also needless in my opinion.

Disclaimer: I am not a radiologist, nor have I had any training in reading CT scans.

So why would I include CT pictures and radiology reports in this book? It is not exactly light or entertaining reading. Well, if you had gone through this journey with my husband, you might understand how frustrating it was that no medical professional hardly ever shared any of this information. It was only years later that I began digging through the reports and scans. I guess you could call me a self-taught learner by necessity and desperation. And determination to find a diagnosis.

Now we will delve into a few other measures that are used to diagnose iNPH. This is the idiopathic NPH or when the NPH doesn't have a known cause. There is also fNPH which is the familial type of NPH which I will discuss at the end of this book.

Disclaimer: All of the CT and MRI images are authentic but I am not a radiologist and no claim is made for an accurate diagnosis from these images.

Figure 9: Tim's CT Scan 12/03/2012

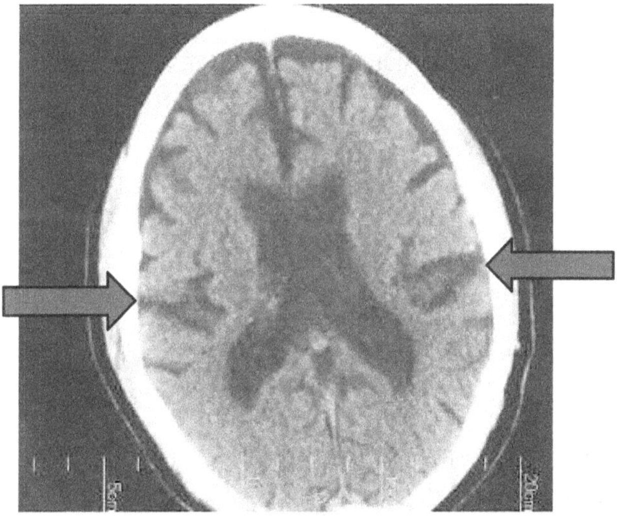

Widened insular cisterns as shown by blue arrows and are a good representation of the iNPH that can respond to treatment.

The Evans Index is a ratio that's used to indirectly assess the condition of the ventricles in patients with Normal Pressure Hydrocephalus (NPH). It is calculated by dividing the maximum width of the frontal horns of the lateral ventricles by the maximum internal diameter of the skull at the same level. The Evans Index is most commonly used in axial CT and MRI images.

I will measure all of the Shunt Brothers CT Scans using the Evans Index when I compare their scans later in the book.

Figure10 : TIM'S CT SCAN: 5/30/2014

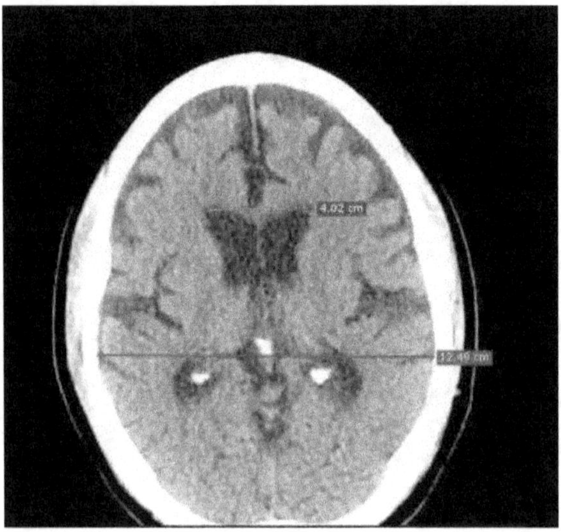

This is a measurement of Tim's CT which demonstrates he met the requirements for ventriculomegaly in 2014. I'm pretty sure no measurements were taken, but it's a pretty easy formula to figure out. You measure the width of the lateral ventricles at their widest and divide by the maximum internal diameter of the skull. The top figure the lateral ventricles measure 4.02 cm and the skull diameter measures 12.40 cm. So 4.02 divided by 12.40 is .32%. Anything greater

than .30 is ventriculomegaly which is enlargement of the ventricles.

Disclaimer:

I am not a radiologist and this is for demonstration purposes only. I'm not sure when the Evans Index came into common use as a measuring tool but CT software allows an untrained individual to attempt to take measurements. I'm not claiming these are exactly accurate or could be used for a diagnosis.

So is any doctor going to dispute that my husband was showing NPH on all of these measures? On one of our last visits to Neurology at KCVA, we were sitting in an examining room talking to a resident. The Chief of Neurology who evidently knew who we were yelled down the hallway so all could hear, "Tell them we can't help them." No documentation of that comment but it was something I never forgot even so many years later. The irony is that it was true. They couldn't help us.

At this time I belonged to a national online group of NPH survivors and those seeking a diagnosis. It was very helpful and the director had been misdiagnosed herself. And she was in her fifties. She advised that it would indeed be impossible to get the diagnosis through Veteran's Affairs. She proved to be right.

I recently showed my normal CT pictures and then my husband's MRI and CT's from 2008 -2014 to my 6 yr old and 10 yr old granddaughters. They were then to tell me if their Grandpa's scans were "good" or "bad". He got 10 bads and 1 good (after shunt placement in 2014.) Pretty smart girls!

I guess the key factor is to get past the initial CT Scan when they tell you it does not show ventriculomegaly (enlarged ventricles). And this happens more than you think would be possible. It happened to 3 of our Shunt Brothers and what it means is you go through more debilitating symptoms for probably several more years. A little knowledge of CT Scans can be a good thing for caretakers. Also, to insist on a lumbar puncture/spinal tap to distinguish this from Alzheimers or Parkinson's disease or just plain old age. Whip out your cell phone and video your loved one before and after. Then a PA or physical therapist cannot decide that there is no improvement and believe me, this will happen as well. And you can always ask for a 3 day spinal tap if there is any doubt about the results.

So that's enough on CT's for now. I will compare some of the brother's scans to see how they compare a little later on. I would like to mention a few more symptoms to look for other than the classic 3 that you always hear about: cognitive problems, balance and magnetic gait, and urinary problems.

Those 3 do not have to be present either at the same time in order to get a diagnosis.

Other Common Symptoms

Tremor

Tremor is common in 40% of NPH patients. In our shunt brothers group we had 3 members who had this symptom. It most commonly appears as involuntary shaking in the hands but can be seen in other parts of the body too. It will most likely be improved after shunt surgery.

Anxiety

Anxiety can present as both physical and/or emotional, and include numbness, tingling, shaking, heart pounding, indigestion as well as several others. Emotionally, patients are impacted by feelings of nervousness, fear of losing control, and an inability to relax. Anxiety is thought to be induced in NPH patients by a decline in the orbitofrontal area.

Personality Changes

These changes include irritability, fatigue, withdrawal, sadness, and an inability to eat or sleep. Brain imaging studies have shown that depression can be associated with right dominant brain dysfunction. Wide scientific evidence confirms association between NPH and psychiatric symptoms. These may include: obsessive compulsive disorder, hallucinations or delusions. Disturbances in executive and memory function predominate. These symptoms would all present with Tim but more on that later. And again, he had some co-morbidities so it is hard to figure it all out.

So these are all symptoms that are overlooked, but you as a caregiver will certainly notice them. Several studies have proven that early detection of the disease will improve outcomes tremendously. They talk about a six month window. I don't think any of the Shunt Brothers were diagnosed that quickly and certainly not my husband. When brain damage occurs it is usually permanent, so oftentimes the cognitive improvement does not return as quickly, although there will be some improvement. There have been numerous studies on the importance of early diagnosis.

A shorter duration of clinical symptoms (e.g. less than 6 months) and the onset of gait difficulty with little or no cognitive impairment also suggests a better prognosis with CSF shunting. Early treatment may also be associated with greater improvement than treatment at later stages of NPH.

One study concludes that patients with an early stage NPH reported at the follow-up an improvement of their symptoms after shunt operation in 65 percent and those with a late stage NPH in 50 percent.

So what prevents patients from receiving early treatment and the right diagnosis?

Maybe the slow onset of symptoms, blame put on other factors causing the symptoms. Ignorance of the disease by our medical professionals. Not performing the crucial tests to diagnose it. Or attributing it to other similar neurological conditions without ruling it out first.

I keep reading that CT scans cannot diagnose NPH by themselves. Yes, ask for an MRI if possible. They can do flow studies and other things CT scans cannot. But the crucial test is the lumbar puncture. It is not "invasive" as I have read. It is no worse that having a blood draw lying on your stomach for awhile. Be sure they do the required tests before and after. It is the best way to nail down a diagnosis because no other dementia will improve this quickly with a large volume CSF tap. The gait problems should disappear. However it only lasts for a short while. A lumbar puncture with fluoroscopy is also a good thing to ask for. And if you don't agree with the results, ask for the 3 day lumbar drain.

Complications of Shunts

11

It seems inevitable that with a human devised device implanted in the brain with various tubing and catheters going in various directions, there might be a few complications. And so it was with the Shunt Brothers.

Studies indicate a complication rate between 20 to 40%. Complications include overdrainage that may cause low-pressure headaches and possibly subdural hygromas as bridging veins tear from ventricular walls and cause "brain bleeds".

We had complications in all 4 of the Shunt Brothers. Sorry to say much of it was due to physician error and the shunt malfunctioning itself.

Tim's complications began soon after the shunt was implanted in December 2014. The neurosurgeon mentioned numerous times about the catheter draining the ventricle being "a little short" but also "it should be ok." Well, it wasn't ok and five months later I was crying in the waiting room because Tim was was no better, in fact he was worse. They did some testing on the shunt including a shunt patency test and shunt series and indeed the catheter was not draining fluid at all. So every month when he had a CT scan and they told us "everything looks good" they basically didn't know what they were talking about. And neither did I because this was before I knew anything about CT scans.

So then we had revision surgery on May 2015 and we were in the "all clear". Except the shunt we had was changing settings whenever Tim was around a strong magnet. I knew this because I would stand behind the Neurosurgeon when he checked the setting and invariably it had changed on its own. That is impossible said the Neurosurgeon but indeed he was proven wrong. I took in a children's toy that had hung on our refrigerator for decades with a strong magnet. Here it is straight from the 1980's.

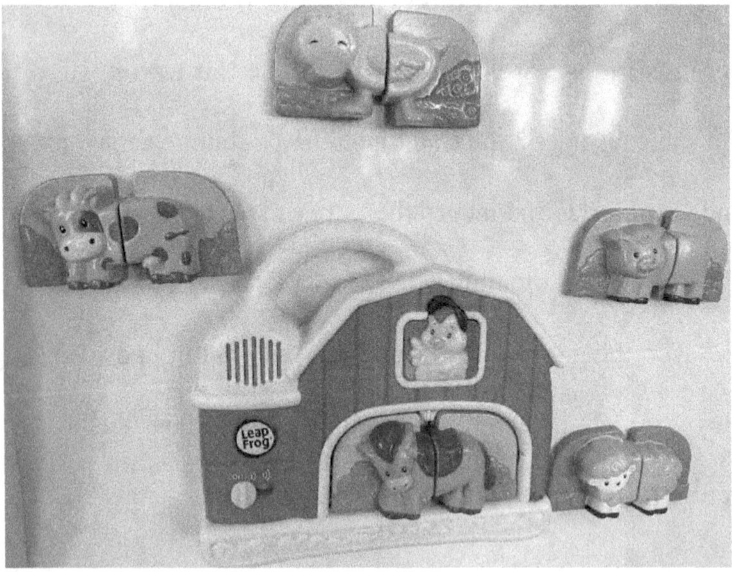

And then I stood behind the Neurosurgeon and watched as he demonstrated the little arrow flip from the lowest to the highest setting. This is very bad for the brain because sudden changes with the shunt's settings can cause all kinds of issues.

So I'm not naming the manufacturer but after a lot of back and forth, they offered to replace the valve. But they were offering the exact same valve with the exact same issues so we said no thanks.

Six months later we had the valve replaced in Oklahoma City at the VA hospital. The neurosurgeon there conveyed that they had a lot of problems with the original valve as well. The new valve has worked quite well for approximately 7 years. So live and learn.

But I forgot one of the most important complications of the original valve. Tim developed hematomas from too much drainage. It landed him in the hospital for several weeks and was a serious issue. The CT done at the time shows a large hematoma on the right side and a smaller one on the left.

We were transferred from Centerpoint in Independence to the KU Medical Center for treatment. This neurosurgeon was into not believing Tim had Normal Pressure Hydrocephalus in the first place. What??? These were my words documented in VA Notes when he was released. We immediately went back to Mayo Clinic for follow-up. Our niece Marsha went with us and was a godsend at this time because Tim was having behavior issues due to shunt malfunction issues. Thank YOU Marsha!!!

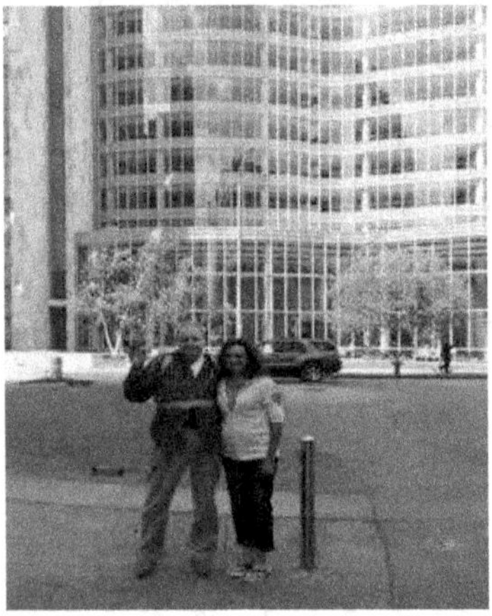

KCVA-

Wife reports that she spoke to Neurosurgeon and he denied that her husband ever had Normal Pressure Hydrocephalus. She reports that she tried to tell the Neurosurgeon the patient was evaluated at Mayo Clinic

and Centerpoint and diagnosed to have Normal Pressure Hydrocephalus. She reports that Neurosurgeon did not accept that conclusion.

I was standing there in total disbelief. This was the Head Neurosurgeon of the largest hospital in the Kansas City area. I tried to explain that I had not made this diagnosis myself, that it had been diagnosed at Centerpoint, confirmed at Mayo Clinic and here we are with a shunt implanted for NPH. Didn't matter, he maintained his position.

Figure 11: TIM'S CT SCAN 8/07/2015 Showing hematoma

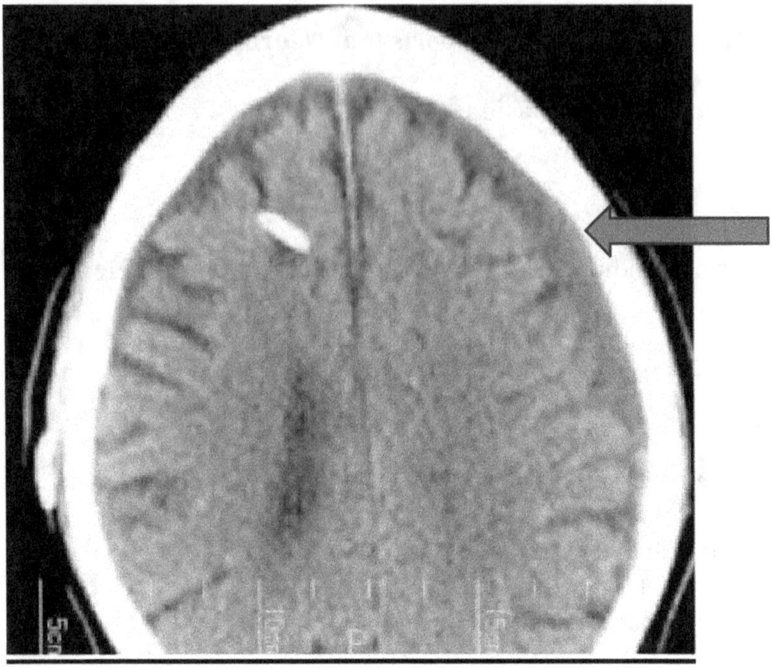

The Blue Arrow is pointing to the area of the hematoma. There is a small amount on the left side too. The white tip is the shunt.

Pat had his shunt surgery in 2021. The Neurosurgeon made the mistake of getting the tubing and catheter into the muscle instead of into the stomach cavity where it drains and is absorbed back into the body. Instead it drained into the abdomen and caused him a lot of pain for several weeks before he had the surgery revised.

Ray had his surgery in January of 2024. He had the setting changed after a few weeks and within two weeks time it had caused a hygroma, or “bleeding on the brain”. Some notes from his daughter Marsha will explain what he experienced:

May 2, 2024- Took dad for a follow-up visit with neurosurgeon. After discussing the progress, we decided to adjust it “1/2 click” to 1.0. His balance has been off, back to taking smaller steps or even stopping and feeling “stuck.” He’s also had quite a few headaches with some being only in the right temple. I spoke to the nurse and was told that’s normal.

May 17, 2024- Routine CT before next visit. The office called and wanted him in the office today for an immediate adjustment. My dad had been having headaches almost nightly or when he gets up in the morning.

June 3, 2024- CT- Everything looks good.

July 9, 2024- Took him for his CT prior to his next follow-up in a few days. We left Christian Hospital and headed for biscuits and gravy breakfast. Forty-five minutes later, I received a call from the nurse asking how quickly we could get to the doctor's office. We quickly finished and headed straight to the office. The doctor, very concerned, explained the CT results and why we were called in. Though we didn't know what caused this drastic change, the shunt had to be put on the lowest possible setting of 2.5 so there was minimal draining. There was a huge blood mass, which pushed his brain over and one ventricle even crossed the midline.

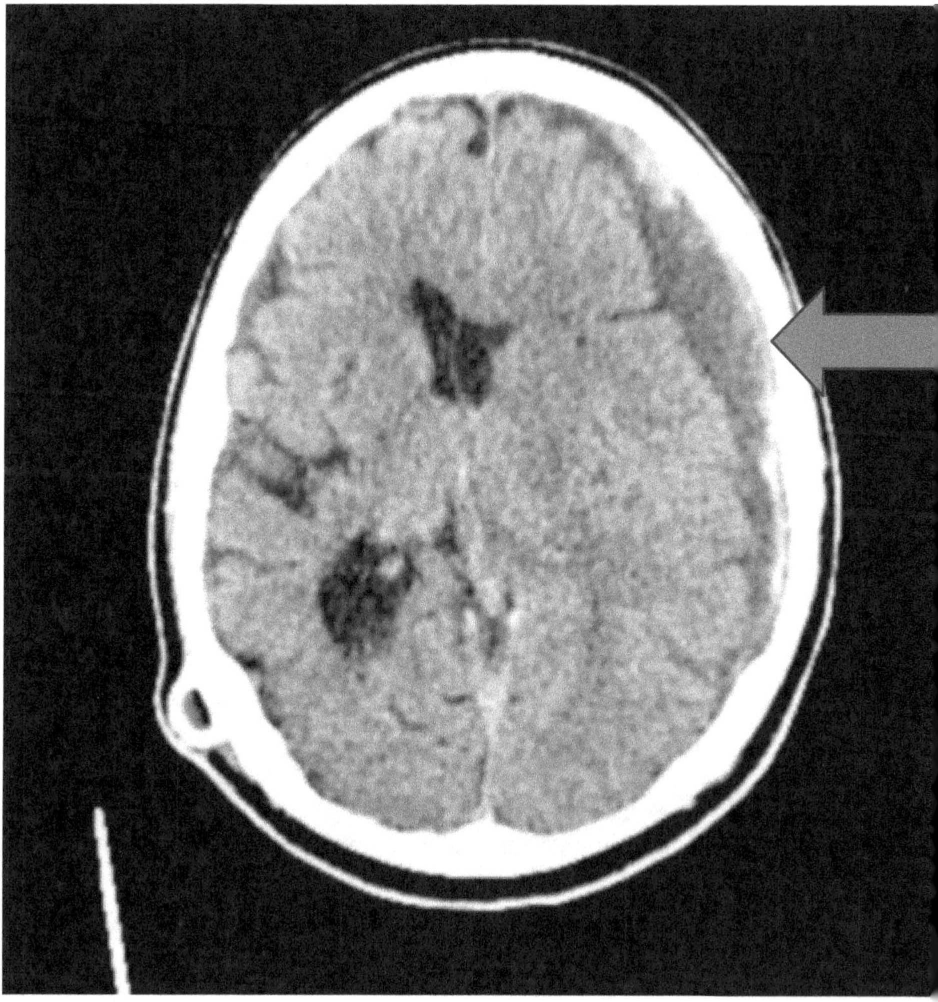

Figure 12: CT scan 7/9/24 of Ray's Hematoma

A couple of days later we had an appointment with a referred colleague who specializes in this type of emergency. He needed to have Middle Meningeal Artery Embolization for his

Chronic Subdural Hematoma. In plain English, it means the shunt was overshunting which shrunk his brain size from excess suctioning. This pulled the brain away from the side and caused the vessels to break and bleed which caused the massive pool of blood.

July 24, 2024-MMA Embolization-

They ran the catheter from his wrist up his arm, across the chest and tried to go up his neck, but was blocked by a carotid artery, so they back tracked and had to go through the groin. When they reached the precise point in the brain, it injected a "glue like substance" to block any further blood flow from pooling. They had difficulty stopping the bleeding but with extra help they were able to stop it. He still faces a twenty percent chance of needing a craniotomy but for now things are going very well.

August 23, 2024-

Took dad for his appointment. The doctor is very pleased with his improvement and recovery. My dad is doing great with all things considered. The headaches are gone! His appetite is great! He's walking great and with no assistance, of any kind, much of the time. He does sleep a lot now whether in his favorite chair, my car, his bedroom chair or his bed. We're told this is a normal side effect.

He's been promoted to a three month follow-up which is pretty cool.

In closing, I really want to thank my aunt and my dad's neurosurgeon for all they both have done. I think his outcome would be drastically different without both of them.

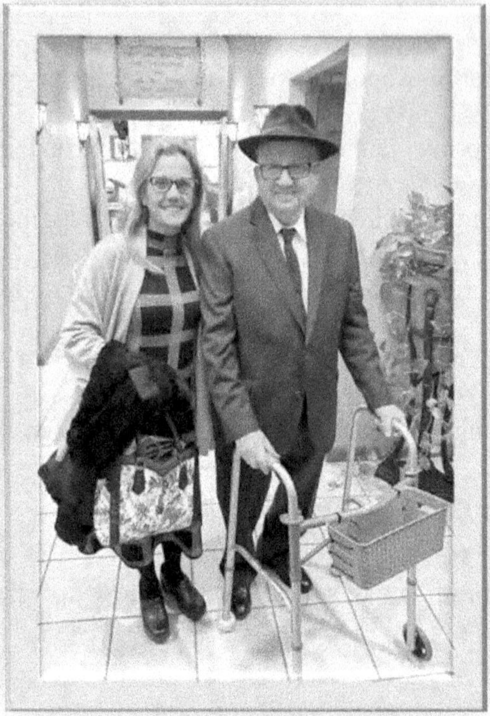

Thank YOU Marsha for your detailed and interesting account. Also your steadfast persistence in getting the diagnosis your dad needed. BRAVO!

Here's a little more from our thread after Ray's surgery to alleviate the hematoma he had developed.

Figure 13: Ray's CT Scan:8/23/24 Before and After MMA Procedure

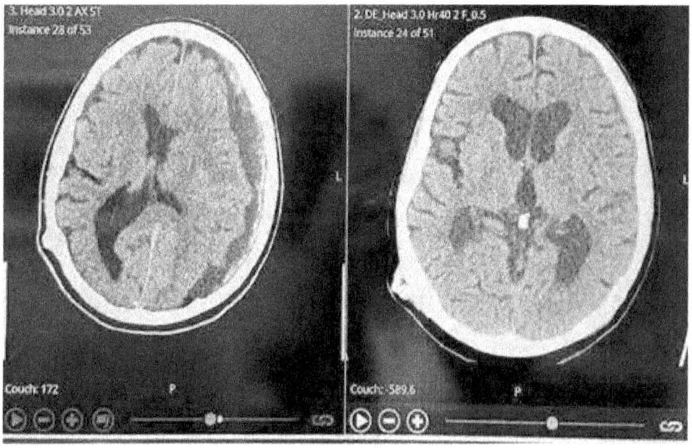

Before *After*

Marsha

I am thrilled to report all of the blood is gone: He's doing really well over all. Some memory issues but my goodness- he's 84 and I have memory issues occasionally. Is a little off balance but catches himself and has not fallen. The thought of turning the shunt back on was discussed. The Dr said he's not seen it before but the very low drainage could possibly be enough for my dad. I suggested we leave things as they are, monitor symptoms and go from there. The Dr was 100% on board. We go back in 3 months as long as things don't change.

It is important not to ignore a headache in the frontal region after shunt surgery because this can be the first sign of overdrainage and/or hematoma/hygroma.

In my research, I came across a couple of things that also might help to prevent overdrainage. One study found that more overdrainage-related complications occur when the initial valve opening is set well below the lumbar puncture CSF opening pressure. A follow-up study showed that setting the valve pressure close to the lumbar puncture opening pressure resulted in less overdrainage.[1]

---

[1] Vivas-Bultrago.,Domingo R. Tripath S., et al Neurol Neurochir Pol. 2020

In NPH valve opening pressure close to lumbar puncture opening pressure decreases overdrainage.

Antigravitational valves appear to reduce the risk of overdrainage, as demonstrated by a randomized double-blind study that reported overdrainage is 7% compared to 43% with programmable valves alone.[2]

One more interesting fact about shunts. We discovered that all five family members had the catheter of their shunt placed 0n the right side of their skull. Is this a coincidence or was there a reason? Here is the answer:

Side Preference

While either side is viable, there's a noted preference for placing the shunt on the right side. This is to minimize risks associated with the dominant hemisphere, which is typically the left side for right-handed individuals, reducing potential complications like speech or motor function issue.

---

[2] Lemiche J. Meier U., Miller C. et al Je Neurol Neurosurg Psychiatry 2013

Safety and efficacy of gravitational shunt valves in patients with iNPH: a pragmatic, randomized, open label multicentre trial.

They are conducting some clinical trials of a new procedure that will not require a shunt. A Yale neurosurgeon is using a minimally invasive approach which involves implanting a device called an eShunt. It is implanted between a vein in the neck and the base of the skull. It allows the CSF to drain into the venous system, or the blood, where it is reabsorbed. I believe they are doing clinical trials at our local KU Med as well. It was not available for our Shunt Brothers, but certainly sounds like a better option Hopefully this will help alleviate all of the shunt complications.

Shunt Adjustments

12

Inevitably at some point you need a shunt adjustment. Sometimes this is not that easy. First their protocols say you must return to the neurosurgeon that put in the shunt. But what if he moved away, retired, got caught in a malpractice suit, or unfortunately passed away? Then you are left begging almost for another NS to take you on and listen to your symptoms. And sometimes they will refuse to even listen to your concerns. It's another struggle, almost as bad as the original diagnosis.

These were actual occurrences with my husband when we sought a shunt adjustment:

He sought an adjustment because the shunt had been turned off due to a hematoma. All of the symptoms had returned in short order but he was still denied. One NS had the shunt manufacturer representative there because he was so concerned about it. He tried to explain all the unknowns of NPH as we are sitting there in his office. The shunt rep seemed to be shaking his head in disbelief.

2. NS#2- He said we would need a report from a physical therapist and a neurologist to get an adjustmment. Most neurologists have a 6 month wait. So we passed.

3. We finally drove to Mayo Clinic with a shunt on virtual off and no one would help. A very nice elderly doctor adjusted the shunt. Totally worth the 500 mile trip.

4. A year later we were in almost the same situation although this time the NS was in Oklahoma City because we went there for a shunt replacement. It was on a very low setting but the

first time back he would not adjust it. Then a few months later we went back with a lot of symptoms and I pretty much insisted we needed it adjusted, so he got mad and moved it 2 settings up. And Tim seemed to do fine on that setting.

It pays to speak up when your loved one needs an adjustment and believe me you will recognize the recurring symptoms that were just relieved by the shunt surgery.

A study from Unfallkrankenhaus Berlin:

One year after shunt placement 80 patients underwent CT scanning and their ventricular size was ascertained using the Evans Index. 80% of the patients showed no postoperative change in the volume of the ventricles and 59% had good to excellent clinical improvements. A moderate reduction in ventricular size was observed in 14% of patients. [3]

---

[3] Meier NH, Mutze S. Acta Neurochir Suppl. 2005

Does the ventricle size change after shunt operation of Normal Pressure Hydrocephalus?

A common scenario when you return to the neurosurgeon to talk about a shunt adjustment due to the reoccurence of the original symptoms is they do a CT scan and come out and say everything looks "fine." But if the ventricle size doesn't change in the majority of shunt surgery patients (80%) then how can they say that with any confidence? It seems like the symptoms reoccuring would be the most important thing to discuss. And if a shunt adjustment is made, you can always look for any signs of overdraining, the most obvious being a new frontal headache. In Appendix 2 there will be a list of other shunt testing that can be done if a shunt malfunction is suspected.

Personality and Psychiatric Changes

13

The longer a person has NPH the more they are at risk for personality changes and development of other psychiatric symptoms. That is because of the damage done by the pressure of the CSF on the frontal lobes. Among NPH symptoms in frontal dominance

Irritability Depression

Increased likelihood of angry outbursts

Disturbances in executive and memory function

Delusions of persecution Mania

Apathy Lowered tolerance

Anxiety Obsessive Compulsive Disorder

Sadly my husband developed almost all of these symptoms over the course of several years. And I was totally in the dark about what was causing them.

He did have "co-morbidities" as doctors like to say. One of them was PTSD from Vietnam. It is probably impossible to send an eighteen year old to fight for their life and not come home with psychological issues because of it. But mostly it was anxiety caused by nightmares, flashbacks, and loud noises. Pretty easy to distinguish from other personality changes.

Around 2004-05, he was hospitalized for PTSD for 3 months and he was retired from his job due to unemployability due to work-related problems. He had worked 22 years at KCVA hospital and received several commendations for his work. He was an excellent carpenter and we have beautiful pieces he built as a hobby. He specialized in cedar chests. He built this cradle for our two children when they were babies.

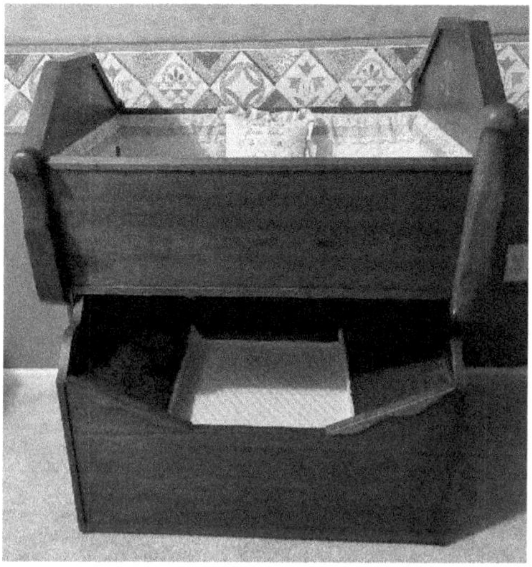

It rocked, it rolled, and had storage underneath!

I won't go into the years we went looking for a diagnosis, as I have already covered that. But a lot of the symptoms mentioned above became problematic even with the anxiety drugs that VA put him on for PTSD.

In the summer of 2014 (still before shunt treatment) he suffered a pretty bad fall from our deck onto the concrete patio and suffered a head injury in the frontal area. A brain injury can also lead to many behavior issues as well. Then after the shunt was placed in 2014, it was another 5 months before it began draining properly and then another year of shunt changing settings before we had it replaced. Finally, he had a stroke in May of 2016. Now with all these issues, it is a complicated case isn't it? I was told that numerous times by different doctors.

Most of the OCD behaviors worsened after the stroke. He had major damage to his thalamus from the stroke and this is what caused it I believe. Later on after a full assessment by VA neurology, he was diagnosed with "probable" vascular dementia.

I will not go into details of the many behavioral problems, but after several short hospital stays and being sent home with the same issues, I tried to get him some longer term help at VA. This turned into quite the journey as I will document along with my support group of sister-in-laws and niece on our chat log. It turned into a two month ordeal. There is a study in Appendix 1 that links NPH presenting as a delusional disorder and leading to dementia.

Part Three: Another Difficult Journey

First Stop: VA Hospital

14

First I called VA for their recommendations. I spoke to a social worker who deals with geriatric patients and she recommended a stay at St. John Hospital, a short term psychiatric hospital in Leavenworth, Kansas that deals with dementia patients. She said just to bring him in by ambulance and VA would transport him. Little did I know I would be met with a lot of resistance. They didn't seem to know anything about the facility. They acted like this had never been requested before. After a lot of discussion , they decided to admit Tim and apply for admission to St. John.

Tim went by ambulance to VA this morning. His physical therapist did all of the arrangements and handled everything so well. Thankful for her help. I thought he would be transferred to St. John in Leavenworth but they admitted him and maybe they will do that tomorrow or Friday.

Kathy

What is wrong with him.

Behavioral issues with dementia and NPH. Delusions and just not normal behavior.

Ann

If he had to get admitted I'm glad it was handled for you, Doreen. This whole thing is stressful enough without that! I hope you can have a little peace tonight and that they will be able to treat him properly. Keep us posted please,I'll share with Clancy. Prayers for you guys! Ann

Marsha

Doing the right thing can be SO DARN HARD. You're amazing and have done so much for him in his best interest. Thank you!

Kathy

I admire you for standing by him through all he has had to deal with. You will get a lot of jewels in your crown. Stay strong. If you need someone to talk to just call. Prayers for you both.

In all fairness, Tim has had excellent care in previous hospitalizations and many awesome, caring nurses and doctors at KCVA. But sadly this was not one of them. He was stuck at the end of a hallway in a small room with a roommate and a sitter and a curtain in between. I would sit at the end of the bed because there was no room anywhere else. I could tell after a day or two that they had his medications wrong as he was becoming more and more agitated. It didn't help that there were a gaggle of nurses right outside the door talking loudly and laughing most of the day. And a poor older man across the hall that kept yelling, "Help me, help me!" If you tried to close the door they would come in and admonish that this was not allowed. When I tried to straighten out Tim's medication list, it was like I was asking for something totally out of line. Sure enough, they had cut his medications way down, and I believe he was going into some withdrawal. I had to work my way up the chain through residents and nurses to finally talk to a doctor who agreed with me and restored the right meds.

The next day the poor man on the other side of the curtain who was almost comatose the whole time began hemorraging from a procedure. I heard them yelling "Code Blue" over the intercom and sure enough, it was Tim's roommate There must have been 15 medical personnel that filled the room. It sounded like they were all yelling in different languages and different dialects. Finally one doctor seemed to take charge and they brought the man back. Thank goodness! But Tim was just about to bolt out of there and the sitter had to literally hold him back. Then they brought out buckets of blood and the smell in that room was making me sick. So I stepped out in the hall and the nurse who I had dealt with before told me I could not stand in the hall.

The hall had been literally full of people just a few hours before. I asked why and he said I might see something on a computer. So I asked to talk to the charge nurse because I was done with dealing with this nurse. She talked to me and immediately removed him from Tim's care. Then we got a new roommate who was homeless and an alcoholic who had fallen and seemingly sleeping it off all day. When he woke up we talked about his medications (he had Nurse #1) and the same thing happened to him. They cut his medications way down and he had only one pain med all day. His leg was swelling and I asked if he needed something for pain. Finally, the nurse checked on him and they discovered his leg was infected and he got some pain meds and an antibiotic. After a couple of days, they were wheeling him out. I hope he has found a better life because he expressed he didn't have much desire to live anymore and he was relatively young. After a few days of all this excitement, I was ready to get Tim out of there, but it didn't seem that they were in too big of a hurry to get him moved. So I started calling St. John myself asking if they had vacancies. Yes, they did they told me. I started putting some pressure on the residents and doctors that I was speaking to and getting nowhere. I got chewed out by one of the residents, but they got the application sent in.

Thank you to Pat and Kathy for the beautiful bouquet. Much love to both of you right back!

The good news on Tim is he's been accepted by St. John in Leavenworth. The bad news is they have a Covid exposure and he probably won't go until Monday. His roommate left and he got a room by the window so that helped. some. Thank you for your love and support as always.

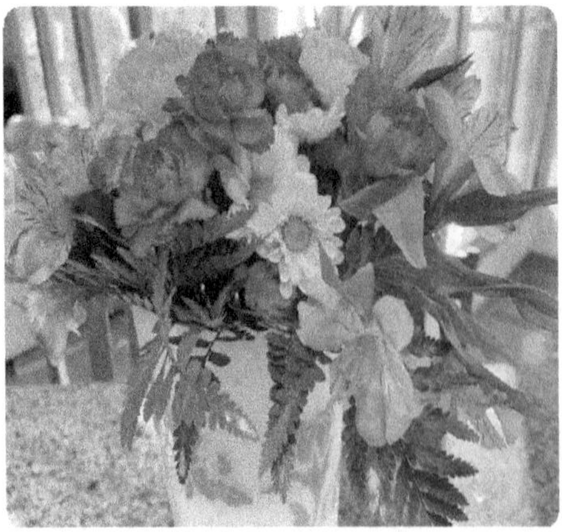

Second Stop: St. John Psychiatric Hospital

15

So after spending two weeks in that environment at VA, Tim finally made it to St. John by ambulance. I was not allowed to go until he was settled in which was a few days.

> I saw Tim yesterday. It's a really small place with only 6 patients. I felt sad about leaving him there and wondering if this was the right decision. But he seems to be tolerating it and they are changing up his meds and monitoring him. He said he'll be there 10-15 days.
>
> I will go back Monday. It's way far up there and I don't like driving thru downtown but I'll survive.
>
> Great news on Ray!

It was quite the contrast! Newly remodeled with private rooms (which I wasn't allowed to see) and a nice meeting room for patients and visitors. It was quite small and with a recent Covid scare, they only had 6 patients. But it was quiet and clean and Tim seemed to be adapting.

They put you on a conference call with the entire team once a week: psychiatrist, social worker, and nurse. They didn't seem to mind at all going through Tim's medications with me, and several needed corrections. They talked to me about new medications and even put Tim on one that I had heard about for delusions (it didn't help him but worth a try.) They were very careful about starting him on a low dose of the psychiatric meds and monitoring his progress.

The downside was it was far for me to drive, so I only saw him once a week. Also, they would not dispense supplements of any kind. That concerned me as an older person needs their calcium, Vitamin D, and Iron.

Tim watches alot of TV and has his favorite shows, but they

didn't provide a TV in the room. That was a real downside to him. And I don't believe he got a whole lot of counseling, physical therapy, or activities. But overall, I was glad he was getting some help. I did feel sad leaving him there and started to question whether this was the right decision. Driving through tears and trying to hold it together on that long drive home to an empty house.

Update on Tim: He's been in the hospital 3 wks now. I saw him Monday and I could see a small positive change. Much calmer and we had a nice conversation for about an hr and a half. Maybe the change in meds is helping. Ironically his roommate at VA told me about 2 meds he takes for hallucinations which I asked for him to try. Hope and pray they help.

On Labor Day, my entire family was here and we all drove up to St. John in my daughter's van to see Dad and Grandpa. I had talked to the social worker and thought the grandchildren could go in (we have four beautiful grand girls). But that was not the case when we got there, as they only let the oldest granddaughter in. (We lied and said she was 16.) They were talking about moving him to a more long term facility because St. John is strictly short term, and he had been there 4 weeks and the psychiatrist felt that he needed more time with the changes in medications to come home. So it was kind of a bittersweet visit. But Tim was glad to see the family. Our sweet granddaughter wrote Grandpa a letter several years ago thanking him for his service in Vietnam.

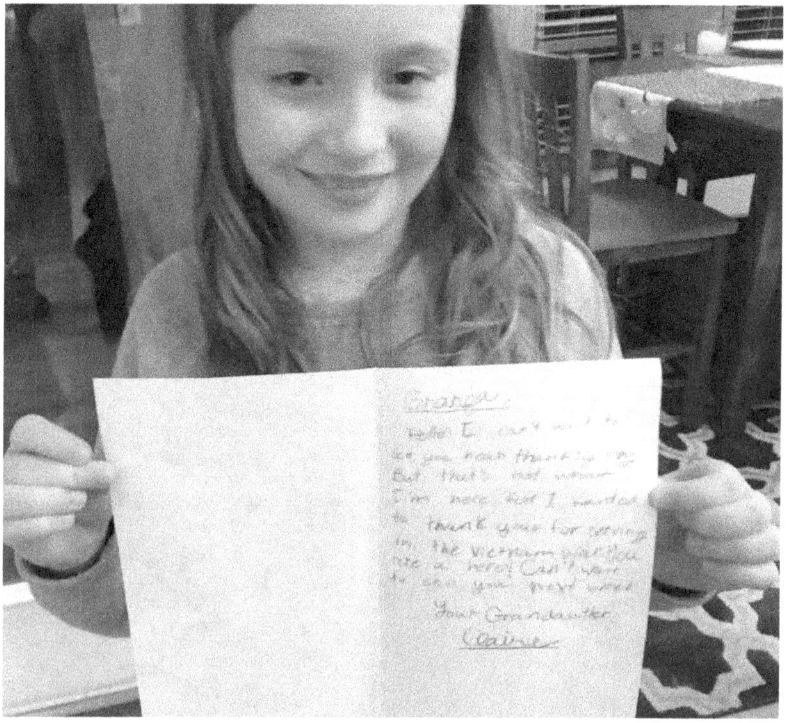

The next week was spent talking to social workers about where Tim would go. It became pretty clear that the VA contracted facilities were few and far between and after being turned down by those that were anywhere near our home, I began calling some myself. They all turned him down, and in speaking to the social worker, she admitted that any VA patient who had been treated for dementia with behavioral problems would probably not be accepted. She said that we have a large population of Baby Boomer patients developing dementia with behavioral issues with no place to go. We do have Missouri Veteran Homes, but they have long waiting lists.

We are still in limbo about where Tim will go. He's still at St. John but the psychiatrist doesn't want him to go home until the delusionary behavior is better. He is eating good and resting alot and being nice to the nurses. Still waiting for the new meds to make a difference. They are trying to get him into a nursing home type setting as they are short term there. Been talking to social workers all week and will go see him tomorrow.Thanks for asking all!

Third Stop: Nursing Home

16

The social worker decided on a facility and within a day they were moving Tim. I had no input and didn't even know where they were taking him. It was a tiny little town even further north in Kansas. I will not name the town but it was so small the silo at the end of a dead end street was the tallest structure in town.

I had to Google the location to even find it. Traveling on numerous two lane unfamiliar roads, I got a little lost the first time. When I saw the sign, population 600, I knew I had arrived. When I drove down this dead-end street, where the silo sits, my heart sank when I saw the nursing home.

I knew before going in that this was not going to work for Tim. And it probably was their last option from VA quite frankly. It was very run down, a little smelly and dirty, and looked like it was built somewhere around the 1950s. The nursing staff seemed to be nice, but they were most definitely understaffed and overwhelmed with the workload. When I saw Tim, I told him I would do whatever I could to get him out of there as soon as I possibly could. And I kept my word.

After speaking my mind a little bit to the VA social worker, she agreed there are not many options for veterans with dementia. Several employees told me they do not keep them very long, especially with behavior issues. For the most part, they cannot be admitted to behavioral health because it is considered "organic." And she said most VA doctors prefer to keep them "in-house." Which is why I was met with so much resistance I suppose. They don't have a long-term treatment center in-house at VA. Perhaps they should.

So after checking out a few private-pay facilities, I decided to bring Tim home. Working through all the paperwork required, he spent two weeks at the facility.

To say we were both glad when he finally got out of there would be an understatement.

Ann

Clancy told me last night, after he talked to you. I couldn't believe it!! I thought it sounded like he would be there a lot longer so that was amazing news! I'm so glad for you and for him that he is calm and I'm sure he loves being back home!

Yes he was ready and so was I. Funny story: Our cat disappeared for about a week and I told him about it in the car coming home. Shortly after he got home he said he could hear meowing coming from the ceiling. After a search of the house, there she was in the top part of the attic and was too scared to jump down. After pulling her down he said, "Now the whole family is home."

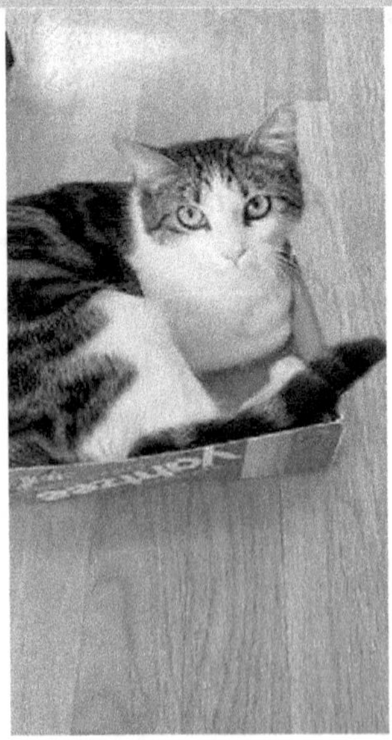

Lessons Learned:

17

1. Speak up always on your loved one's behalf. When you're dealing with a lot of residents especially at VA, ask to speak to the hospitalist in charge of your loved one's care.
2. A psychiatric hospital can be a good thing because it gives any new psychiatric medication time to work. I knew very little about 2nd generation anti-psychotic medications, but I was pleased to find out that they do work to help calm OCD behaviors.

3. The behavioral aspects of long term untreated NPH can be attributed to frontal lobe damage and is similar to dementia-related behavior.
4. There's always light at the end of any tunnel!
5. You are stronger than you think you are!

Part Four: Co-Existing

Conditions in the Shunt Brothers

Co-Existing Conditions That May Contribute to the Development of NPH

18

There are several conditions that have been identified that either contribute to the development of iNPH or appear in larger numbers in the people with iNPH in case studies. Among these are:

Cardiovascular disease

Vascular disease

Diabetes mellitus

Hyperlipidemia (High cholesterol)

Hypertension (High blood pressure)

Essential tremor

Peripheral neuropathy

Cerebrovascular disease

Peripheral vascular disease

Many of these are inherited and they appear in large numbers in the elderly population anyways, I'm sure. But I thought it would be interesting to canvass the Shunt Brothers and see how many coinciding conditions we come up with. I'll start with my husband Tim:

Vascular disease- Total blockage of left carotid artery

Stroke (caused by blood clot) and eye stroke

Essential tremor (controlled)

Peripheral neuropathy

Hyperlipidemia (controlled)

Hypertension (controlled)

Cerebrovascular disease-Vascular dementia

(hypometabolism)

Cardiovascular disease- Atrial Fibrillation, Bradycardia (pacemaker)

Pat:

Cardiovascular disease- Heart attack due to blockage, bypass surgery

Vascular disease: Stent in aorta from stomach, stent in aorta from heart

Peripheral vascular disease

Clancy:

Peripheral vascular disease (stent surgery)

Peripheral neuropathy

Essential tremor (controlled)

Ray Sr:

Diabetes

Cardiovascular disease

Ray Jr:

Diabetes

Cardiovascular disease: Atrial Fibrillation

Essential tremor (controlled)

Hypertension

Hyperlipidemia

So we have 4 out of 5 with cardiovascular disease, 3 out of 5 with vascular disease, 3 out of 5 with essential tremor and 2 out of 5 with diabetes.

Seems like more than a coincidence. Here is some research on the contribution these diseases and their statistical occurrence in case studies with patients with iNPH.

Vascular risk factors in iNPH-

- **Our findings confirm that patients with iNPH have more vascular risk factors and lack the protective factors present in the general population. Almost 25% of cases of iNPH may be explained by vascular risk factors. Hypertension, cerebrovascular and peripheral vascular disease were also overrepresented in iNPH.[4]**

Diabetes is associated with familial iNPH: a case-control comparison with family members

[4] Hanna Israelsson, Bo Carlberg, Carlsten Wikkelson, Katarina Laurell, Babar Kahlon, Goran Leijon, Anders Elklund, Jan Malm Neurology 2017

Diabetes is associated with fNPH and a possible risk factor for fNPH. Diabetes could contribute to the pathogenesis of iNPH/fNPH.

- **Diabetes (32% vs 14%) , arterial hypertension (65% vs 43%) cardiac insufficiency (16% vs 2%) and depressive symptoms (32% vs 8%) were overrepresented among the probable fNPH patients compared to their non-iNPH relatives.[5]**

<u>Heritable essential tremor-idiopathic normal pressure hydrocephalus</u>

This new autosomal dominant genetic disorder known as essential tremor-idiopathic normal pressure hydrocephalus was detected in a family with 15 members

---

[5] Joel Rasanen et al Fluids Barriers CNS 2020

effected with ET, of whom 3 of them in the second generation developed iNPH.[6]

While genetic predisposition is a significant factor, environmental influences can interact with an individual's genetic makeup to exacerbate or mitigate the dietary habits, and overall lifestyle choices.

Genetic Predisposition and Environmental Interactions

19

Traumatic Brain Injury

Traumatic Brain Injury is one of the well-documented risk factors for developing secondary NPH. Repetitive

---

[6] Zhang J. et al Am J Genet A. 2008

head trauma, even when not severe, can lead to the accumulation of damage over time, potentially contributing to the pathophysiology of iNPH.

Cardiovascular Health

Cardiovascular health is another crucial environmental factor. Conditions such as hypertension, diabetes, and hyperlipidemia, which are influenced by lifestyle and environmental factors, have been associated with the development of iNPH. Cardiovascular health can affect cerebral blood flow and intracranial pressure regulation, potentially leading to the symptoms observed in iNPH patients.

In Appendix 1 is a synopsis of how NPH can cause frontal lobe dysfunction which manifests as dementia leading to a

delusional disorder. A study is presented that proves 2nd generational antipsychotics are successful in treating it.

In Appendix 2 the differences between NPH and Alzheimer's, Parkinson's and other dementias is explored.

Part Five:

The Shunt Brothers Share Their CT and MRI Scans

A big THANK YOU to the Shunt Brothers for sharing their scans. I appreciate it so much and will be using them to make some comparisons and contrasts. Maybe you will understand how they can also be used to come to a misdiagnosis. Or learn about a term for a diagnostic tool called DESH (Disproportionately Enlarged Subarachnoid-space Hydrocephalus).

We will first make some just straight up comparisons. Keep in mind that these CT scans were taken at different times in their journey. Some were done days before diagnosis, some were years before the diagnosis, and one was taken a few months after shunt placement.

Is This Ventriculomegaly?

20

Figure 14: Ray's CT Scan: 6/9/22

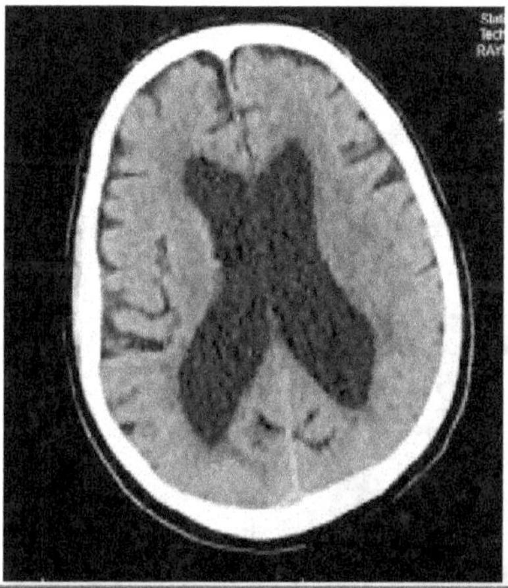

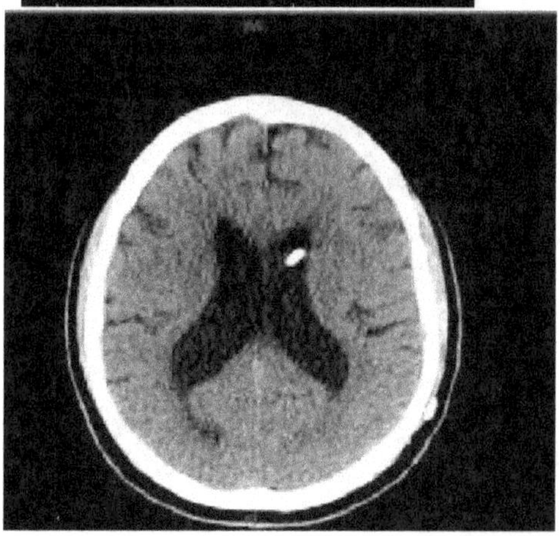

Figure 15: Pat's CT Scan: 1/5/24

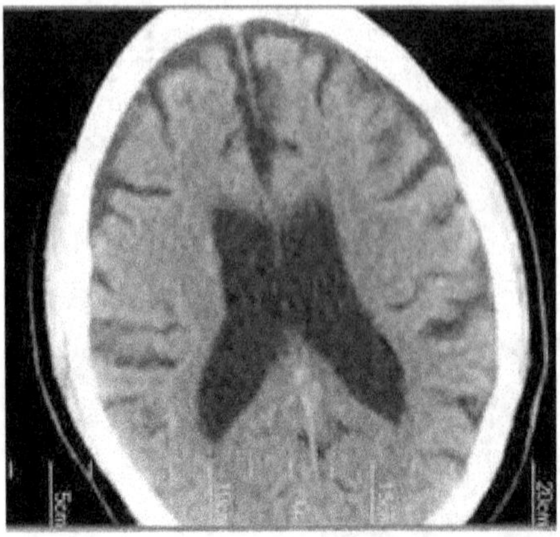

Figure 16: Tim's CT Scan: 5/30/2014

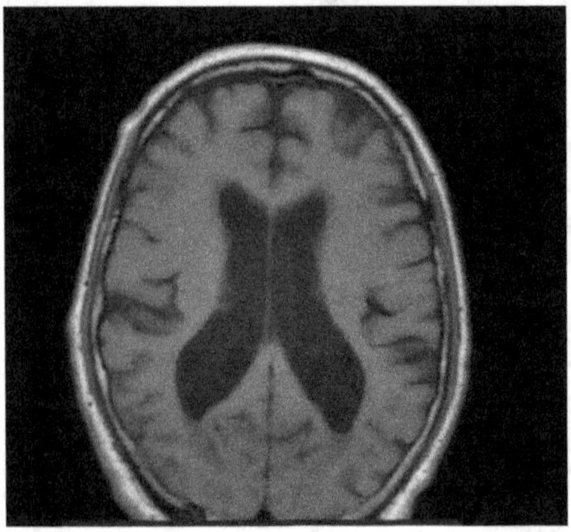

Figure 17: Clancy's MRI: 1/5/24

It is astonishing how similar these scans are isn't it? It would be hard to tell one brother from the other using these scans. It would seem to this author that they inherited this disease.

Anatomy of a Misdiagnosis

21

Now we will demonstrate how to make a misdiagnosis in a few easy steps. This probably happens every day in the U.S., but it sounds like many other countries grapple with this problem as well. It is estimated that Japan only diagnoses about 10 percent of their population who have NPH. And they have done quite a bit of the research into the disease. The story begins with Ray Jr. who was transported to the wrong hospital OSF Saint Anthony's Health Center in Alton, Illinois. He had suffered a bad fall and they immediately did a CT scan. Then they found out his insurance would not be accepted at this facility. So he was sent home and was doing so poorly, he was sent by ambulance to Alton Memorial Hospital. They repeated the CT scan and he was dismissed with a referral to see a neurologist.

I have received the CT scans and reports from his daughter Marsha. I thought it would be interesting to compare them,

The first CT scan was taken at Saint Anthony's Health Center where Ray was mistakenly taken. The second CT scan was taken at Alton Memorial Hospital after he was taken there later in the day. You would expect them to have the same appearance and with just a few minor differences, they do look identical.

What is extremely interesting is the CT report that came with the scan. Here is an excerpt from the wrong hospital, St. Anthony's Health Center:

IMPRESSION:

Enlargement of the lateral and 3rd ventricles out of proportion to degree of volume loss, potentially representative of more central cerebral atrophy, with Evans index of 0.36 (elevated even when adjusted for age and gender) NORMAL PRESSURE HYDROCEPHALUS

should be entertained in the appropriate clinical context. Otherwise, no acute intracranial process with chronic findings as above.

Translation for the non-medical jargon folks: The Evans Index is an important criteria for NPH as anything over .30 is considered elevated. Also the "appropriate clinical context" is probably the same symptoms that Ray presented with and are the hallmarks of NPH: Cognitive difficulties, urinary issues, being unbalanced with many falls, and unsteady gait.

The second report from Alton Memorial I did not receive, but I don't believe NPH was mentioned. He had been treated here numerous times and they never diagnosed it. The only diagnosis I heard was "mild fluid on the brain." It struck me as odd knowing the family history of NPH.

After his Alton Memorial Hospital visit, sadly these concerns were dismissed. He was referred to an outside neurologist and even with the family history discussed, there were 2 brothers diagnosed with NPH at this time, it would be another year and a half of troubling symptoms before he was diagnosed and treated.

Figure 18: Ray's CT Scan St. Anthony's 6/9/22

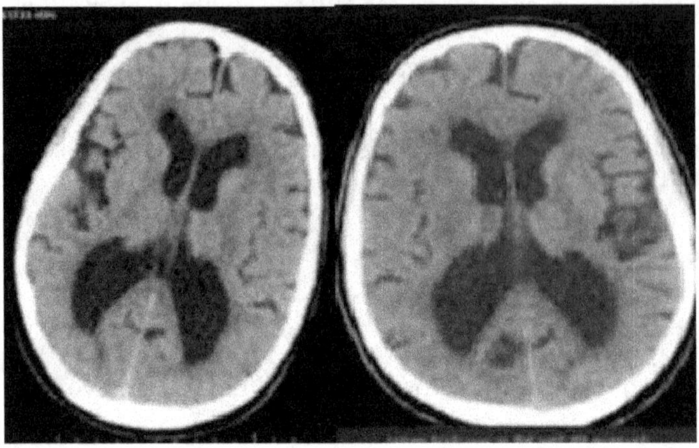

Figure 19: Ray's CT Scan 6/9/22 Alton Hospital

So close, but yet so far away from getting the correct diagnosis. If only the neurologist had listened to Ray's family members about the brothers already diagnosed and did at least the basics like a spinal tap, maybe Ray could have gotten the correct diagnosis.

Contrasting the Shunt Brother's scans with the Evans Index and DESH

22

A refresher on the measurement of the Evans Index: It is the largest diameter of the frontal horns of the lateral ventricles divided by the diameter of the internal skull on the same plane. A value greater than 0.3 for the Evans Index is the only essential morphologic criterion of probable iNPH as reported in the journal Neurosurgery and the Japanese guidelines.

Figure 20: Pat's CT Scan: 9/16/21

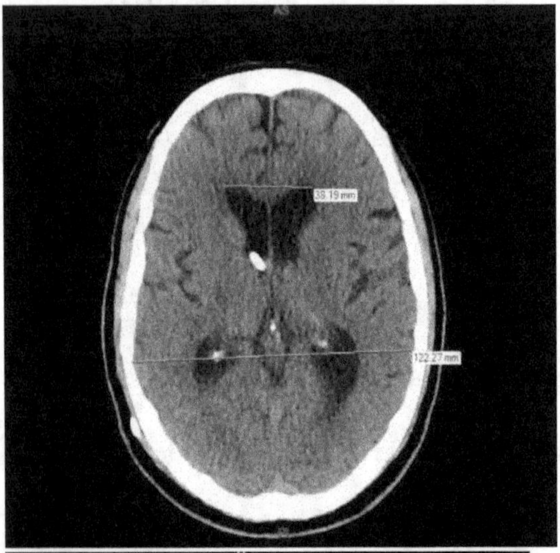

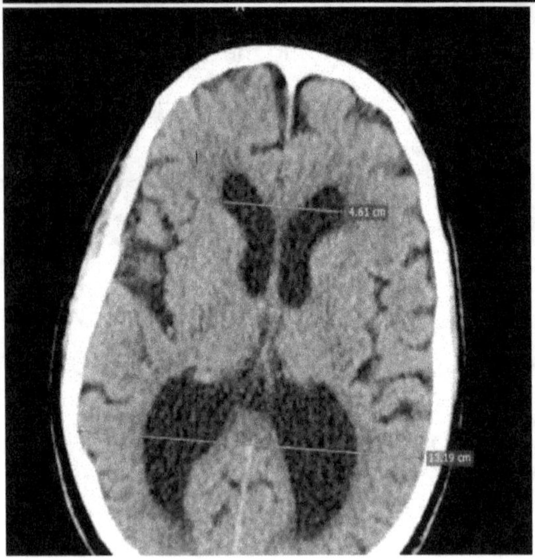

Figure 21: Ray's CT Scan: 9/28/22

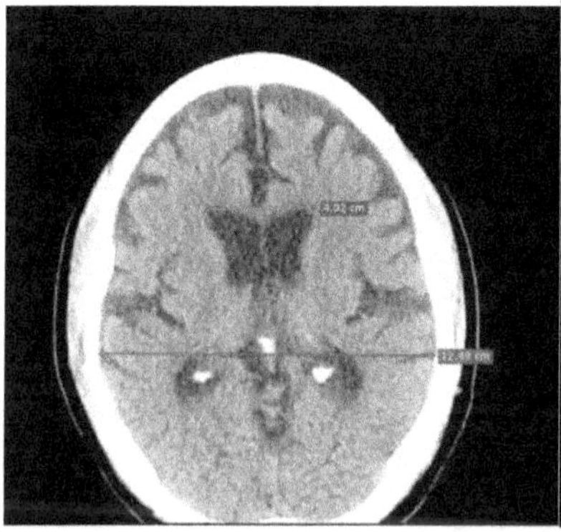

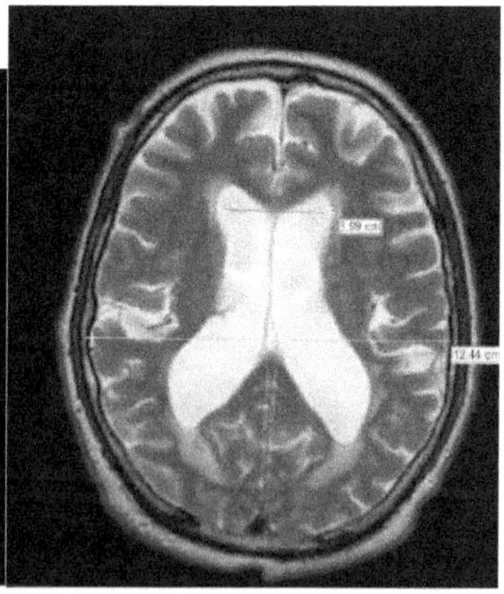

Figure 22: Tim's CT Scan 5/30/14 **Figure 23: Clancy's MRI 1/5/24**

So the Evans Index is calculated like this for the Shunt Brothers:

Figure 1: Pat:- 38.19 mm divided by 122.27 mm = .31%

Figure 2: Ray Jr.- 4.61 cm divided by 13.19 cm= .34%

Figure 3: Tim- 4.02 cm divided by 12.49 cm=.32%

Figure 4: Clancy-3.99 cm divided by 12.44= .32%

Interpretation of the Evans Index:

.20-.25 Normal

.25-.30 Possible or Early Ventriculomegaly

>.30 Ventriculomegaly

So we have 4 Shunt Brothers with definite ventriculomegaly. I don't presume to be a trained radiologist and these scans are just to illustrate how these measurements are taken. I do believe it is commonly used to interpret CT and MRI scans, so you are not out of line to ask for the Evans Index measurement.

Another measurement that is increasingly used is called "DESH". It stands for Disproportionately Enlarged Subarachnoid Space Hydrocephalus. Basically it requires Dilated Sylvian Fissures, Evans Index over .30 and tight convexity of the sulci at the vertex. I will attempt to point out these measurements on a few of the Shunt Brothers scans to illustrate. Again, this is only for illustration purposes and no claim is made for their radiological accuracy.

Now let's examine several CT images of the Shunt Brothers and see if they meet any of the requirements for DESH. The blue arrows are pointing to Dilated Sylvian fissures which are visible pockets of CSF fluid. All of these scans show dilated fissures which is a requirement for DESH. The other lines are measuring the Evans Index which was discussed previously. Again, all of these scans showed an elevated Evans Index score.

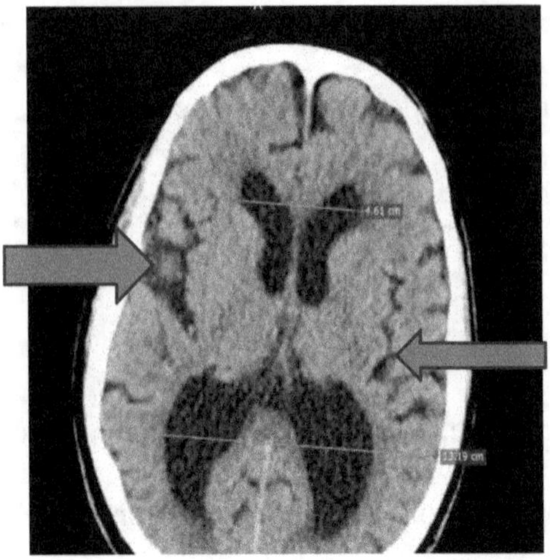

Figure 24: Ray's CT Scan 6/9/22: EI:.34

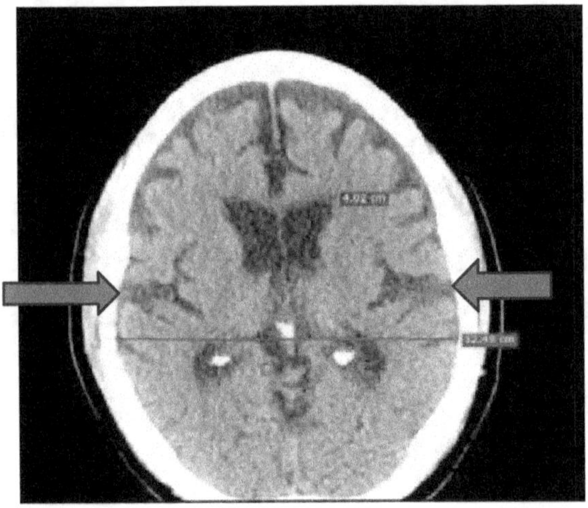

Figure 25: Tim's CT Scan 5/30/14: EI:32

These meet two of the requirements for the DESH score. They all have Evans Index scores <.30 and the Sylvian fissures are all visibly dilated. The 3rd requirement is tight convexity of the sulci at the vertex. Since this is rather difficult to differentiate on a CT scan, I am going to demonstrate it's appearance on an MRI Scan. This is also a subjective score as no measurements are taken.

Disclaimer: These images are shared from authentic CT and MRI images but no claim is made for their acuuracy of diagnosis and are used only for comparison purposes.

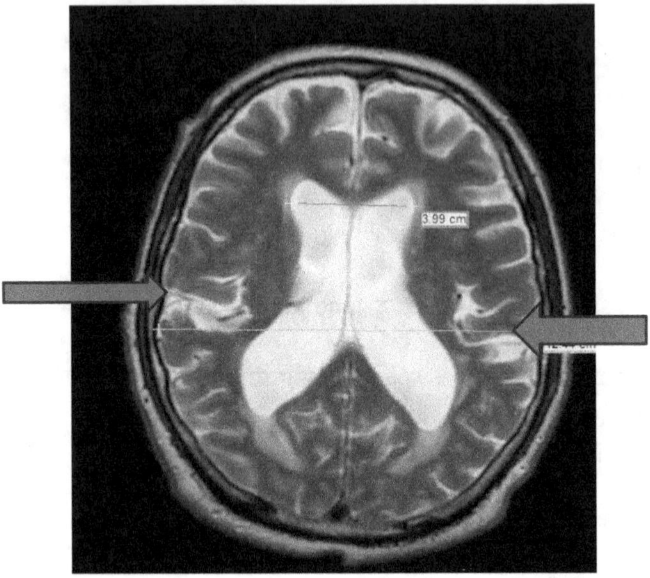

Figure 26: Clancy's MRI 1/5/24

The Evans Index score is .32 and the blue arrows point to the dilated Sylvian Fissures.

The CSF is visible in the frontal lobes. This is what is causing the symptoms Clancy was having. He was diagnosed the next day January 6, 2024.

Figure 27: Clancy's MRI: 1/5/24

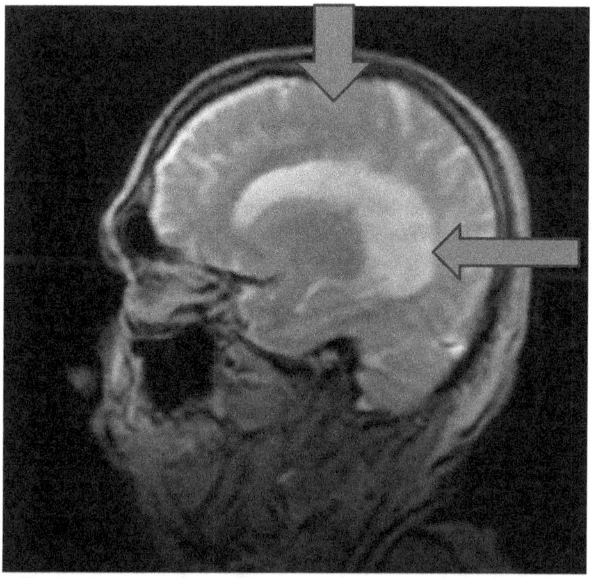

He has an Evans Index of .32 and Dilated Sylvian Fissures. Tight Convexity of the sulci at the vertex on top. Ventriculomegaly of the temporal horns of the lateral ventricles.

So with all three requirements met, he has met the qualification for the DESH score. In his report, they mentioned disproportionate enlargement of the lateral ventricles, acute callosal angle and sulcul crowding at the cerbral cortex. Again, he was diagnosed with NPH the next day 1/6/24.

Disclaimer: I am not a trained radiologist and these scans and measurements are for illustrative purposes only. No claims are made for their accuracy or reliability for a diagnosis.

A Comparison of Two Shunt Brothers MRI's: Which one has NPH?

23

This is a comparison of Tim's MRI in 2008 and Clancy's MRI in 2024. I'm sure there has been some advancement in diagnostic measures in the ensuing years, but the fact is many patients are still being misdiagnosed with all the new knowledge in 2024. This was proven by the Shunt Brothers and their delays in the correct diagnosis. But I will delve into that a little later.

3-pl T2 FGRE (This is the code for the slices taken with the `MRI)

This is an MRI with contrast to highlight the areas of CSF accumulation. Clancy is showing excess CSF in the frontal lobes, while Tim has excess CSF all across the surface of the vertex, or the top of the brain.

Figure 28: Clancy's MRI: 1/5/24

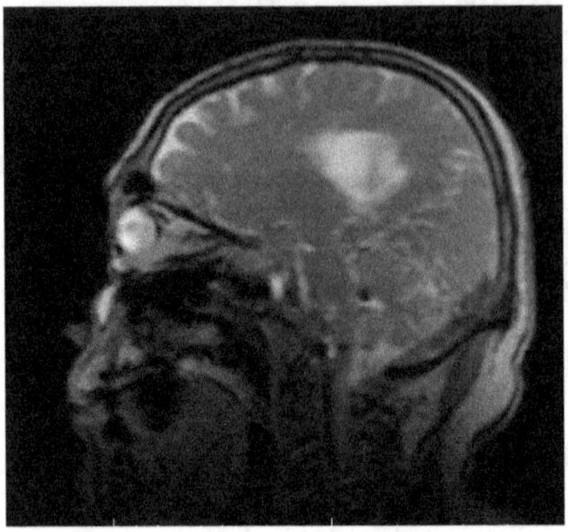

Figure 29: Tim's MRI: 4/17/08

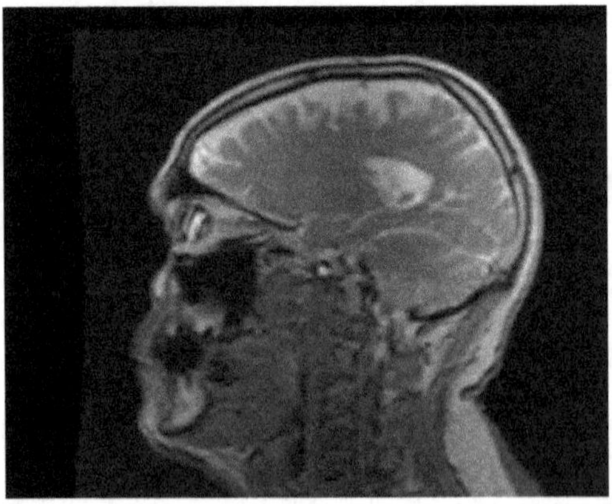

Figure 30: Clancy's MRI: 1/5/24

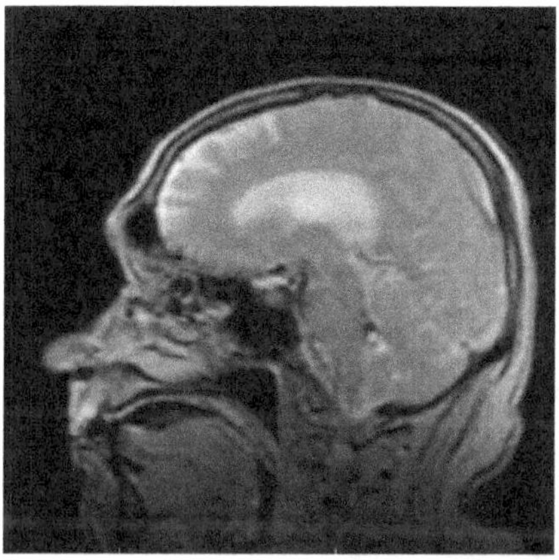

Figure 31: Tim's MRI: 4/17/08

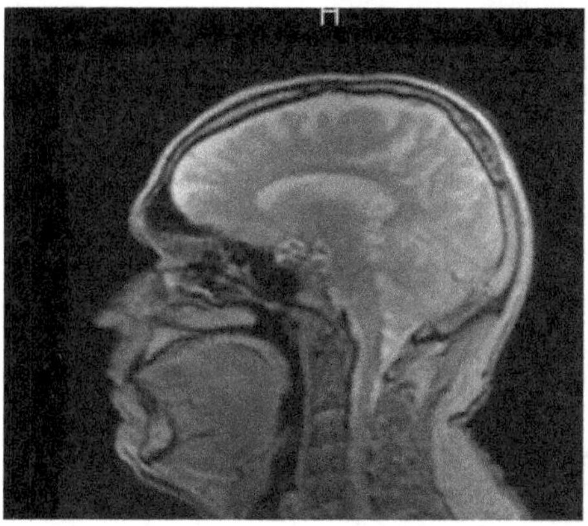

A better image of the CSF build-up in the frontal lobes, and all across the surface of the brain in Tim's. Also we see the fluid build up in the frontal lobes of Clancy's MRI.

Figure 32: Clancy's MRI: 1/5/24

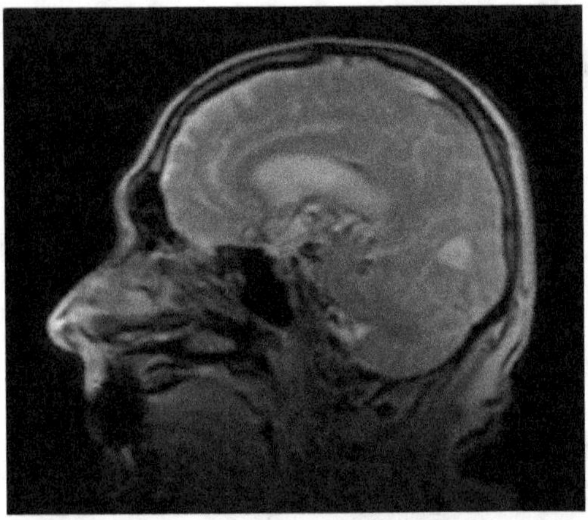

Figure 33: Tim's MRI: 4/17/08

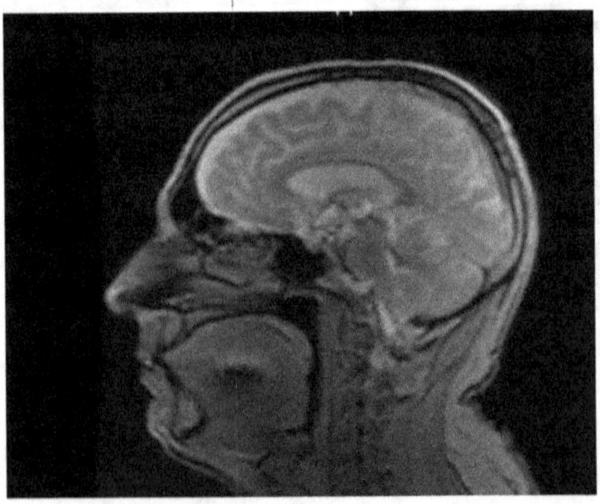

Clancy has more ventricular enlargement in the temporal horns of the ventricles while Tim has more overall CSF accumulation in the sulci (folds of the brain).

Figure 34: Clancy's MRI: 1/5/24

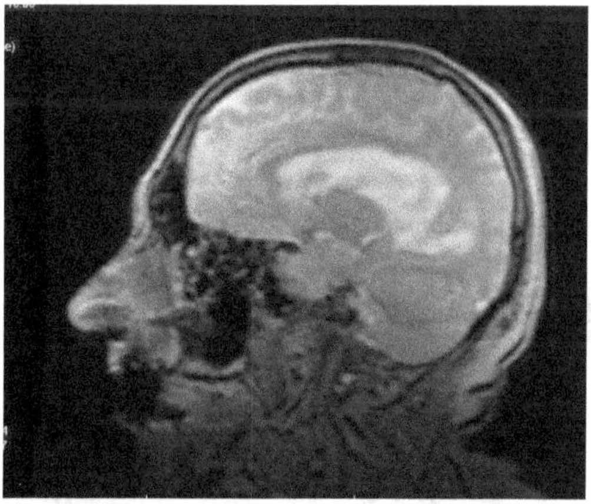

Figure 35: Tim's MRI 4/17/08

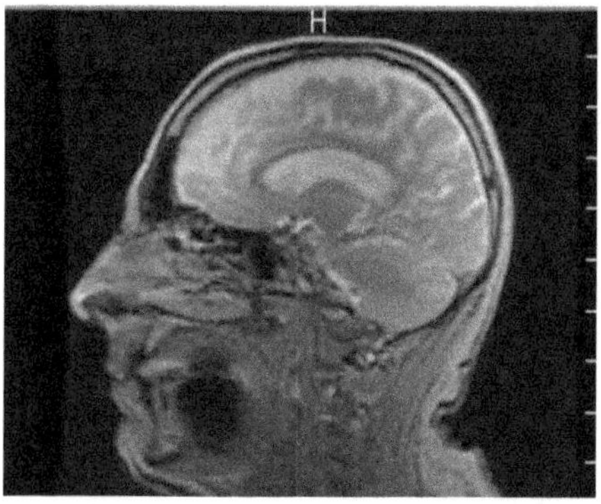

A good view of the ventricular enlargement of the temporal horns of the lateral ventricles in Clancy's view. In Tim's the excess fluid in the frontal lobes and across the vertex is quite visible.

These are images from the MRIs which show the ventricular enlargement and excess fluid in the sulci.

Figure 36:Clancy's MRI: 1/5/24 **Figure 37: Tim's MRI 4/17/08**

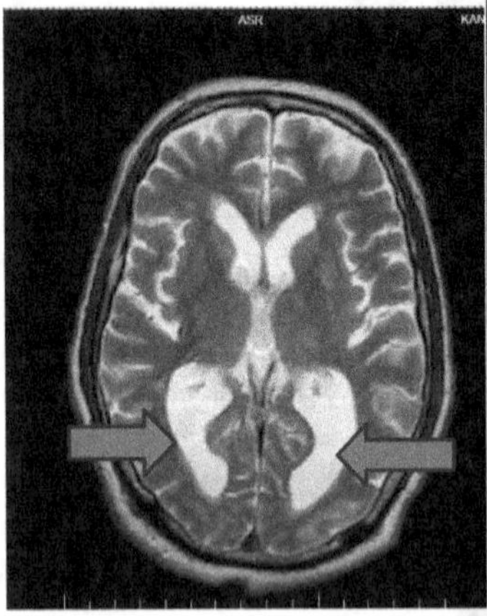

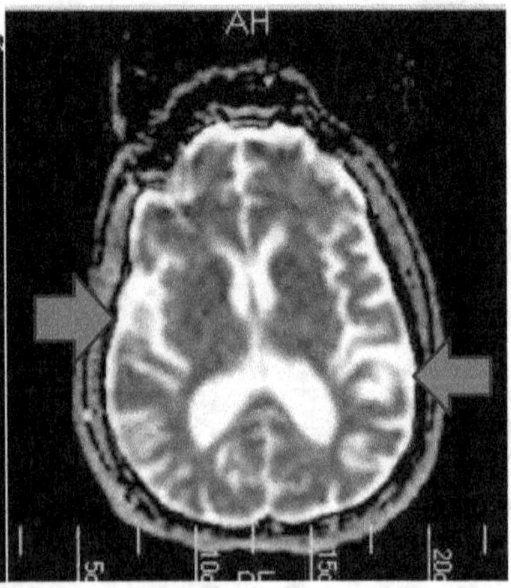

This shows the temporal horns of the lateral ventricles enlarged in Clancy's view and the enlarged Sylvian fissures in Tim's. (blue arrows)

So to answer my own question, they both had normal pressure hydrocephalus.

The difference was Clancy was diagnosed the very next day and received a shunt about a month and a half later. Tim on the other hand, did not receive a diagnosis and went through six more years of symptoms and CT scans every other year and no one figured it out. Sure, they are better at diagnosing in recent years, but the other three brothers still went through years of symptoms and delays in treatment. If it hadn't been for our persistent caretakers bringing up the family history, I'm not so sure they would have been diagnosed. This is unacceptable and the main reason for this book.

Disclaimer: I am not a radiologist and these comparisons are for illustration only and should not be used to make a medical diagnosis.

Comparing White Matter Changes in Two Shunt Brothers MRI's

24

This refers to visible alterations in the white matter near the ventricles specifically caused by CSF leaking out of the ventricles and into the surrounding brain tissue through the ependymal lining. It is caused by increased pressure within the ventricles and is commonly seen in normal pressure hydrocephalus. It appears as hyperintensities on brain imaging and especially MRI scans. On MRI scans the affected white matter appears brighter on T2-weighted images indicating increased fluid content.The presence of periventricular white matter changes, especially when accompanied by enlarged ventricles, can be a significant clue for diagnosing NPH. It oftentimes presents as a "halo" around the ventricles. Here are two MRI scans from two of our Shunt Brothers showing this phenomenon.

Figure 38: Pat's MRI Scan 2/14/22

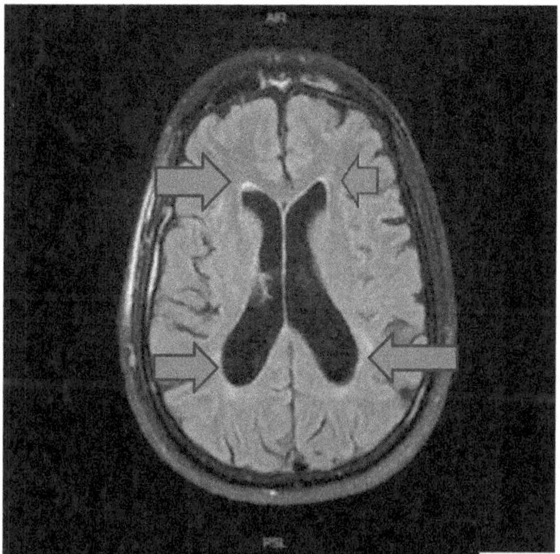

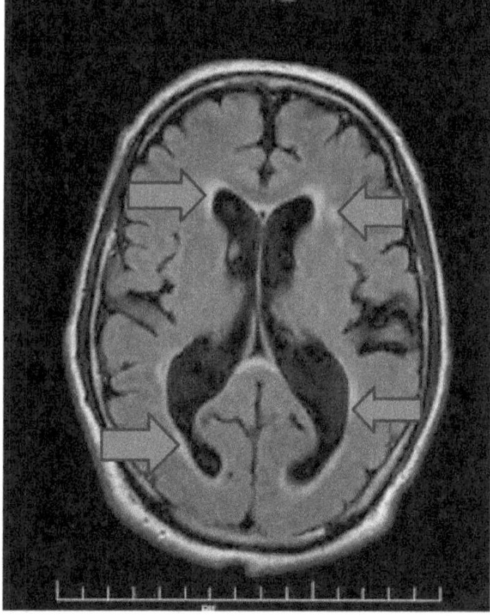

Figure 39: Clancy's MRI 1/5/24

Blue Arrows are pointing out hyperdensities of white matter

One might ask why all these diagnostic measures are important. Well for one thing, after decades of misdiagnosis, there are tools to help determine if someone has the signs of NPH on CT Scans and MRI's. It is certainly true that any of these measures must be corroborated with the clinical signs: gait problems, frequent falls, cognitive issues, and urinary problems. But all too often these signs are dismissed as "normal aging" or "early dementia." In our current medical system, you must go to a primary care doctor most of the time for a referral to any type of specialist. So if you have symptoms but are never referred to a neurologist, you can go years with no diagnosis. Also, there is no guarantee the neurologist will diagnose you as our Shunt Brothers stories prove.

To recap a little of their stories:

Tim- His first CT scan was actually in 2002. The report only states he had "many falls." Then as his condition worsened he had an MRI in 2008, and CT scans every other year after that: 2010, 2012, and 2014. So it took approximately 12 years for the correct diagnosis. And we did indeed see 7 neurologists all in one year when he turned 65 and could use Medicare.

Pat- Complaining of memory issues in 2019. Went to see neurologist with no diagnosis. In 2021 went to primary care with all 3 clinical signs. His wife brought up the family history and 2 family members with shunts for NPH. He referred him to neurosurgeon and then to a neurologist for the diagnosis. Received the shunt in 2021. So approximately 2 years for the diagnosis.

Clancy- Feeling off balance in 2018, shifting from foot to foot at work. He saw a podiatrist and primary care doctor when all clinical signs were causing issues. He first saw a neurologist in 2023 and received a diagnosis of low B-12 not NPH. After a fall in early 2024 and ER visit, he was diagnosed with NPH. His wife, Ann, repeated the story numerous times of the now 3 family members who had received shunts for NPH and were doing well. He received the shunt in February of 2024. So approximately 6 years for the diagnosis.

Ray- Hospitalized 8 times beginning in 2016 with confusion and weakness. When Covid-19 came along he would be diagnosed numerous times with it, but Marsha, his daughter, would bring up the family history because he was also exhibiting the clinical signs of NPH. He eventually got a diagnosis in 2024 and the shunt in January at the age of 84. So approximately 8 years for the diagnosis.

I should point out that nearly all of the medical professionals consulted would not believe that this condition could be inherited. But due to the tenacity of their caregivers, they got the correct diagnosis after telling the family history. Perhaps there are more families out there with similar stories.

Horror Movie Mask or Ventriculomegaly?

25

I have seen the eyes of a Horror Movie Mask compared to the ventricles of a person with NPH. I promise once you see it, it's hard to forget. Maybe just another tool to recognize ventriculomegaly for us non-medical people.

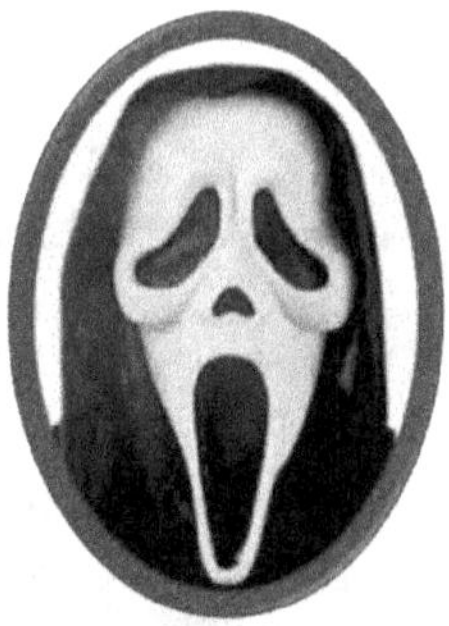

Which Shunt Brother has the best Horror Movie Eyes?

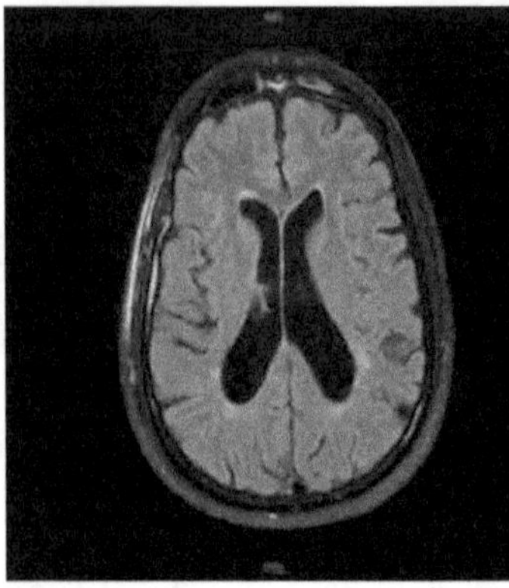

Figure 40: Pat's MRI 2/14/22

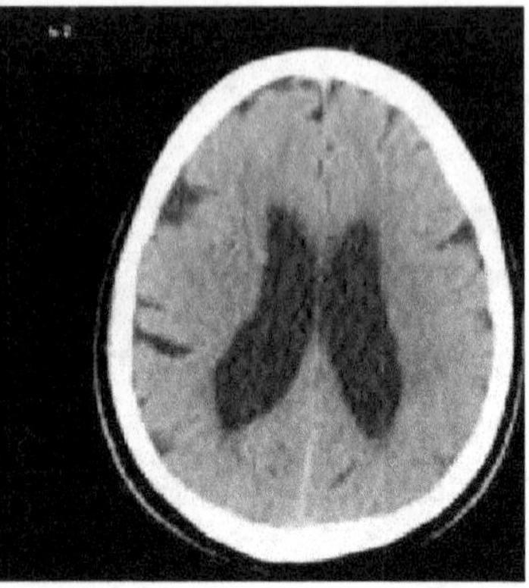

Figure 41: Clancy's CT 1/5/24

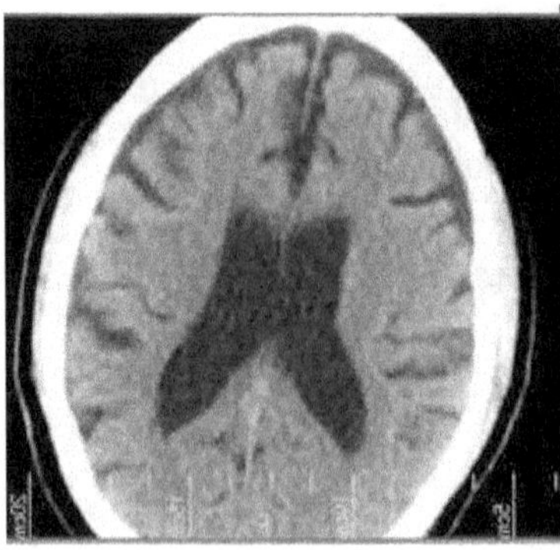

Figure 42: Tim's CT 5/30/14

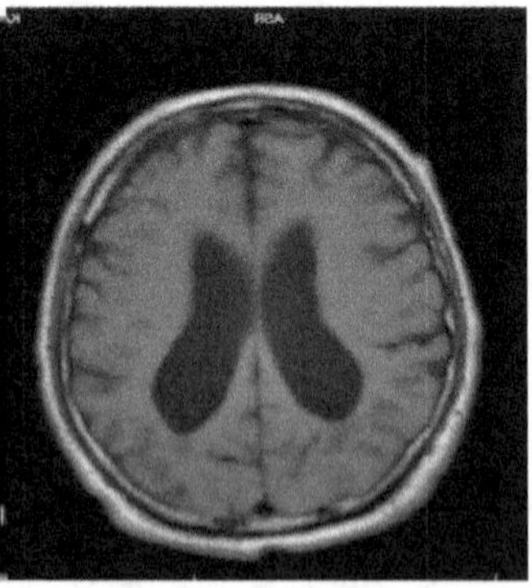

Figure 43: Ray's MRI 4/28/17

Yes, I can see the Horror movie mask ventricles in all of these. Remember, they were all eventually diagnosed, but some had to wait longer than others. I don't know how scientific this is, but it sure is easy to remember and apply. Who wins the best Horror movie mask ventricle contest? I think it was Ray.

Part Six

The History of Normal Pressure Hydrocephalus And Genetic Components of Familial NPH

The Discovery of Normal Pressure Hydrocephalus

26

Dr. Salomon Hakim is considered to be the first to identify Normal Pressure Hydrocephalus as a treatable condition. This was way back in 1957 in Bogota, Columbia and he spent 7 years formulating his hypothesis. In March of 1964 he published a thesis on the condition.
The 50th Anniversary of the recognition of NPH was commemorated on March 10, 1964.

So this condition is not relatively "new" as I have read. It has been identified for 60 years. Today treating NPH is an accepted practice. Diagnosing NPH is an an inexact science as all of the Shunt Brothers can testify to.

So Beware Baby Boomers: A diagnosis of Parkinson's disease, Various Dementias or Alzheimer's is devastating to patients and families as no good treatments are available. However sometimes that diagnosis is wrong as NPH is very treatable and usually gets good results.

Decades after Dr. Hakim's research, his story remains largely unknown and untold. Many people suffering from NPH remain misdiagnosed or undiagnosed to this day by the general medical community. That is what this story is all about.

Fast forward to 1992 to 2022 when a Yale Medical School faculty member suffered the same baffling symptoms of NPH for 10 years. It was diagnosed erroneously as cerebral atrophy and/or Parkinson's disease. I find it extremely interesting that even practicing doctors and a Yale faculty member are misdiagnosed just like us common laypeople. You would think with their access to all the latest medical research, collaboration with colleagues, and medical expertise, this would not happen. But it does. I mentioned the kidney specialist whose story inspired me to dig a little deeper into my husband's misdiagnosis. It was actually a liver specialist who finally diagnosed him and gave him back some of his life. This Yale Medical School faculty member initiated a survey after recognizing the lack of awareness of NPH by physicians. He interviewed 166 practicing physicians who graduated from 50 American and 33 foreign medical schools using a 10 point questionnaire. Almost one third of the physicians had never heard of NPH, One fifth had learned of NPH in medical school and about half learned of it after medical school. Because there were insufficient physicians in this survey from 1986 to 2005, they recruited 118 additional physicians from the 20 Yale Medical School graduating classes from 1986 through 2005. Two thirds of them had learned of NPH in Medical School, and one fourth during residency and fellowship. Seven percent had never heard of NPH.

The Evidence of Familial NPH

27

It's mighty unusual for five family members to come down with the same "rare" condition and for it not to be inherited. But in all of the Shunt Brothers the hereditary possibility was discounted. One neurologist said it could be "environmental" but he declined to name what those factors might be. Upon a little research, it is found that other countries and in the U.S. have identified families with inherited NPH and they are close to identifying the genes responsible for it. Wouldn't it be exciting if family members could one day be tested for these genetic factors and perhaps avoid going through what these brothers went through? Especially since you can have the disease for a long time before even any symptoms appear and early detection seems to be key in successful outcomes. First, I will identify some families in other countries. It has recently been reported in Japan in 2011, and Canada in 2012 and in the

United Kingdom. There is also a family history of shunting in 5% of patients with NPH in Finland. So familial NPH or fNPH may exist in clinically important numbers. Finally a case study that was performed in the USA at Yale, Harvard, and other hospitals and institutions.

So let's explore the familial cases which have been identified over the years. I am using NIH and PubMed for most of these examples. I am just going to summarize these case studies, but I will also put in Appendix 6 the entire list of the sources they came from if you are interested in reading the entire article. Then I will identify the genetic factors that they are studying which may be identified as the hereditary cause of familial normal pressure hydrocephalus or fNPH.

1. **United Kingdom-** We report two sisters with NPH who lived together their entire lives and whose natural history might provide insights into genetic and environmental mechanisms underlying this disorder. Both patients were in

their early seventies, single, had similar daily habits and hypertension. No other family members had NPH.

They both underwent shunt placement and showed improvement documented by history and neuropsychological assessment. No environmental factors that might have influenced the development of NPH were identified.

2. Japan- We report a large family with 4 patients with elderly onset of NPH in three generations. All of them had cognitive impairments, gait disturbance and urinary problems along with normal pressure of cerebrospinal fluid. Their brain MRI showed enlargement of the ventricles and a disproportional narrowing of the subarachnoid space and cortical sulci at the high convexity of the cerebrum, which are the features of iNPH on MRI. The family interview also disclosed an additional 4 patients who were suspected as having NPH in an autosomal fashion.

This is the first family report to show a large family with NPH patients in three generations.

3. Finland- We characterize a potential subgroup of iNPH in a nation-wide Finnish cohort of 375 shunt-operated iNPH patients. The patients were questionaired and phone-interviewed, whether they have relatives with either diagnosed iNPH or disease-related symptomatology. Then pedigrees of all families with more than one iNPH-case were drawn. Eighteen patients (4.8%) from 12 separate pedigrees had at least one shunt-operated relative whereas 42 patients (11%) had relatives with two or more triad symptoms. This study described a familial entity of iNPH offering a novel approach to discover the potential genetic characteristics of iNPH.

4. Sweden- This is a case of two identical twins who were both diagnosed with idiopathic normal pressure hydrocephalus. They both experienced the triad of symptoms and both received a ventriculoperitoneal shunt. Unfortunately, one of the twins passed away before they could do any genetic study to see if they carried the same genes that might be responsible for the disease. The number of familial NPH cases has increased over recent years and it is important to make DNA analysis in future cases of familial NPH.

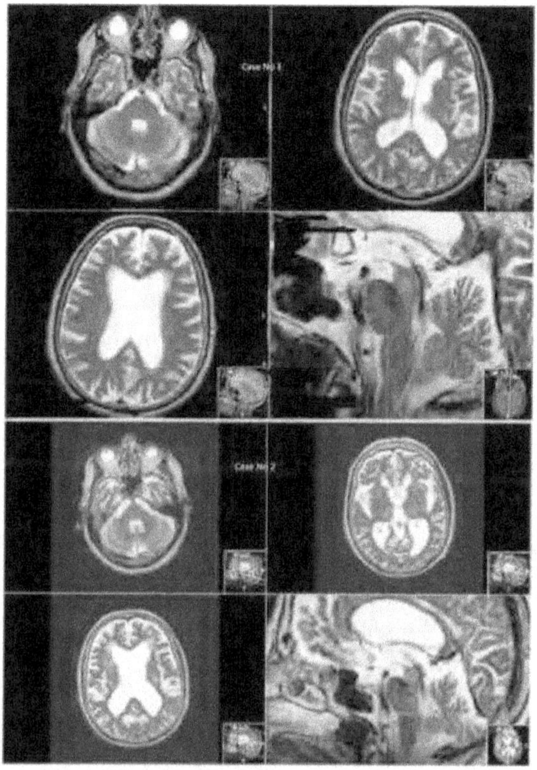

Figure 44: MRI Images of identical twin sister with iNPH

5. Canada- This was case-control family study of the iNPH symptom triad among the relatives identified from a cohort of patients undergoing CSF diversion.

It also presents a novel well-characterized familial case of iNPH. The family study and novel familial case suggest familial aggregation of NPH. Confirmation of heritability may allow identification of individuals at high risk for iNPH and early intervention.

6. USA- A novel case series of 8 familial idiopathic normal pressure hydrocephalus patients. All novel familial NPH patients exhibited improvement following shunt treatment. They also reviewed literature-based evidence for inheritance of iNPH in 22 pedigrees. Analysis of the 30 total fNPH cases reported is highly suggestive of an autosomal dominant mechanism of inheritance.

7. USA- A novel case series of five male members of a Midwest family from Kansas City, Missouri. Four living brothers and their father were diagnosed and received shunts in 1980, 2014, 2021, and two in 2024. Author's note: Just kidding, this is our family and no case study has ever been done, but certainly one would be warranted. Especially since the mere notion of inheritability was discounted with every brother by numerous neurologists and neurosurgeons.

Now for the case reports which explored specific genes. Without getting too technical because I'm far from an expert on genetics, I have researched the cases presented so far and will include their country of origin and important findings. To see the full chronological list please see Appendix 7. I also include a glossary of genetic terms associated with familial NPH in Appendix 5.

From what I have learned, fNPH develops in an autosomal dominant inheritance way. This is caused

when a mutated gene from one parent is enough to cause the condition in a child. Only one copy of the mutated gene is required and the child has a 50% chance of inheriting the mutated gene.

What are the mutated genes? They are also called a "loss of function" variant. They disrupt the function of a protein-coding gene. There is also a "nonsense mutation" which is a DNA change that causes a cell to stop making a protein before it is complete. Another term is "copy number loss", which is also a genetic alteration where a segment of DNA, including 1 or more genes is removed from a chromosone.

Now for the genes and case studies with country of origin:

1. SFMBT1 gene-

Japan- A case study where half of the ventriculomegaly cases (enlarged ventricles) had a copy number loss with the SFMBT1 gene.

Japan- A case study concluding that an alteration in SFMBT1 gene may be a risk for iNPH.

Finland, Norway- Copy number loss in Intron 2 of SFMBT1 among patients with iNPH. It provides further evidence of its role in iNPH.

2. C90RF72 gene-Finland- Analysis of the C90RF72 expansion should be considered for those with probable iNPH presenting with frontal atrophy and severe psychiatric symptoms.

3. CWH43, SFMBT1, DNAH14, CFAP43

United States- Variants in specific genes may contribute to NPH.

Congenital factors are primary contributors to the CWH43 related clinical syndrome.

4. AK9 gene-

United States- Mutations in AK9 and other genes affecting ependymal cells in NPH. (ependymal cells line the ventricles and help regulate CSF).

5. SLCO1A2 gene-

> Finland- A large study that identified new genetic variants associated with NPH. One gene, SLCO1A2 in the microvascular system is intriguing given the heavy comorbidities of NPH.

So it seems a little obvious that the familial form of NPH has been identified for quite a few years. Most of the case studies seem to come from Japan, Finland, Canada, and the United States. Familial NPH has some unique characteristics, is often misdiagnosed, and the earlier it is treated, the better the outcome. I have been moved and saddened to hear the stories of the Shunt Brothers. I knew bits and pieces, but didn't know their complete stories. This was a whole lot of suffering and I know that firsthand by what my husband Tim went through. And why do they keep saying they haven't identified any genetic factors? Again, it seems the Japanese are way ahead of the curve in identifying the SPMBTI and CFAP43 gene and testing with knock-out mice. Knock-out mice are genetically modified lab mice that have one or more genes intentionally "knocked out" or inactivated. Look in APPENDIX 7 for a cool picture of these mice. And the large scale Genome-Wide Association Study from the University of Eastern Finland identified significant variants associated with NPH in six different loci. One gene is associated with vascular comorbidities of NPH.

A few things that I did learn from the research into familial NPH:

- The symptomology is often more severe in fNPH and there is a prevalence of the complete triad of symptoms presenting themselves: magnetic gait, urinary problems, and cognitive decline. This was certainly the case in all four Shunt Brothers.
- The response to shunt surgery is usually remarkably effective. And so it was with all the brothers. Amazing improvement.
- There is almost always a delay in diagnosis as these symptoms are not recognized as NPH or attributed to various other causes. This delay in diagnosis is usually years and the damage to the brain occurs in this time period.
- Imaging can show ventriculomegaly before any of the worst symptoms present themselves. I will share some of the Shunt Brother's imaging to prove this. It is also proven by research.

- Frontal lobe damage occurs the longer the diagnosis takes. This is directly involved in the development of gait disorders, urinary issues, and cognitive decline. It can also manifest itself in psychiatric and behavioral changes.
- Cardiovascular risk factors and subsequent vascular disease development may contribute to the development of fNPH.
- Familial iNPH may be clinically more aggressive than the sporadic iNPH.
- The last large Genome-Wide Association Study from Eastern Finland gives those suffering from familial type NPH some hope that more large scale research will be done into the genetic factors.

Part Seven: Grok

Giving Artificial Intelligence a Chance

To Grok 2 or not to Grok 2, That is the Question

28

So I have been reading about this amazing tool called Grok 2 available on X. Not promoting the site, but I heard you can upload any medical image and get an interpretation that might be pretty accurate. So I thought it might be fun to upload the Shunt Brothers CT scans and MRI's and see what happens. These scans were used to make the final diagnosis of NPH, although of course they considered the clinical signs as well.

So here we go:

The first scan I put up was one of Ray Jr's. from 12/21/23 which was just a few weeks before he got his diagnosis and shunt surgery. Here is our conversation on Grok 2.

Case 1: Ray

← Grok 2 new

What does this CT scan show?

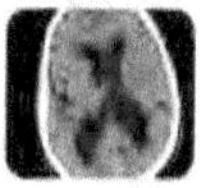

Answer

This CT scan shows a brain with significant abnormalities. The scan reveals:

- **Hypodense areas** (darker regions) which typically indicate fluid accumulation, necrosis, or less dense tissue compared to normal brain tissue.
- **Hyperdense areas** (lighter regions) which could represent hemorrhage, calcifications, or contrast uptake in enhanced scans.

Given the appearance, this could be indicative of:

- **Brain Tumor**: The pattern might suggest a mass effect with surrounding edema.
- **Stroke**: Hemorrhagic or ischemic changes could present this way.
- **Abscess or Infection**: These can cause similar imaging patterns due to tissue destruction and fluid accumulation.

For a definitive diagnosis, correlation with clinical symptoms, patient history, and possibly further imaging or biopsy would be necessary.

The patient has all of the clinical symptoms and has already had a lumbar puncture with marked improvement. So

Show more

Answer

Based on the information provided, if a patient has the classic triad of symptoms associated with Normal Pressure Hydrocephalus (NPH) gait disturbance, cognitive

impairment (dementia), and urinary incontinence—and has shown marked improvement after a lumbar puncture, it increases the likelihood of NPH. The clinical improvement following the removal of cerebrospinal fluid (CSF) via lumbar puncture is often used as a diagnostic indicator for NPH, suggesting that the symptoms might be due to the accumulation of C

Well I'm glad it wasn't a brain tumor, stroke, or abscess or infection. Grok 2 seems to be right on about the importance of clinical symptoms and also the importance of lumbar puncture to confirm a diagnosis.

Next we will explore one of Clancy's MRI views. This was done during the night on Jan. 5, 2024, the night before he was diagnosed on Jan. 6, 2024.

Case 2: Clancy

Grok 2 new

Are the ventricles enlarged in this MRI?

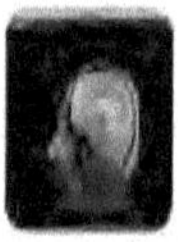

Answer

From the MRI image provided, it's difficult to definitively state if the ventricles are enlarged without clinical correlation or comparison to previous scans. However, they do not appear significantly larger than expected for an adult brain. For a precise diagnosis, a radiologist and clinical context would be necessary.

It's already been analyzed by a radiologist and these are not normal sized ventricles. This patient has NPH.

Answer

Given the radiologist's analysis and your mention of Normal Pressure Hydrocephalus (NPH), the ventricles in this MRI are indeed enlarged, consistent with the condition where the ventricles expand despite normal cerebrospinal fluid pressure. This enlargement is a key feature of NPH.

So just like trained radiologists and neurologists, obvious NPH can be missed on imaging. Just ask our Shunt Brothers.

Next is Tim's CT scan from May 30, 2014. This was the year he was diagnosed and the last CT image it was based upon.

Case 3: Tim

Are there any abnormalities in this ct scan?

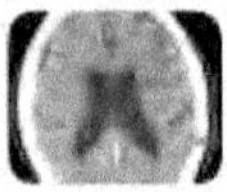

Answer

Based on the CT scan image provided, there appears to be an area of increased density in the left hemisphere, which could suggest a possible abnormality such as a hemorrhage or a mass lesion. However, without clinical correlation and additional imaging, a definitive diagnosis cannot be made. Always consult with a radiologist or a medical professional for an accurate interpretation.

Could this be excess CSF in the correct clinical context?

Answer

In the context of imaging findings, the appearance of excess cerebrospinal fluid (CSF) on a CT scan typically suggests a condition where there's an abnormal accumulation of CSF. This can be due to a variety of reasons including:

1. **Hydrocephalus**: This is an increase in volume of CSF within the cerebral ventricles due to various reasons such as obstruction in CSF flow, reduced absorption, or overproduction.

Case 4: Pat

← Grok 2 new

What are the highlighted areas around the ventricles in this MRI?

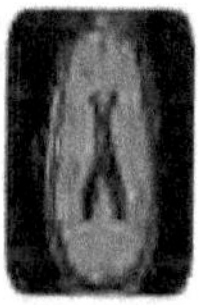

Answer

The highlighted areas around the ventricles in this MRI scan are likely the periventricular white matter regions. These areas are often of interest in MRI scans due to their association with various neurological conditions, including multiple sclerosis, where lesions in the white matter can appear as hyperintense (bright) spots on MRI images.

← Grok 2 new

It appears in 2 brothers MRI scans both of whom have NPH. No other neurological condition.

Answer

If you are observing MRI scans from two brothers who have been diagnosed with Normal Pressure Hydrocephalus (NPH) and you are referring to the "halo effect" or periventricular hyperintensities

I guess the biggest lesson to learn here is if you ask the right questions, you might get the right answers. All of these were way off-base to start with, but I guess that's understandable to a degree because they are not perusing an entire sequence of scans, and they don't have the patient in a clinical setting. Still, it is frightening how many times in the scenario of a neurologist with the CT or MRI scans and a patient with symptoms, no diagnosis is made.

Acknowledgement: Thanks to xAI's Grok for research assistance.

Grok Responds: Familial Cases and Misdiagnosis

29

Would a family of 5 brothers with 4 receiving shunts due to NPH be an unusual occurrence?

Answer

Yes, a family of 5 brothers where 4 have received shunts due to Normal Pressure Hydrocephalus (NPH) would be an unusual occurrence. NPH, particularly in its familial form with autosomal-dominant inheritance, is rare. While there are documented cases of familial NPH, having such a high incidence within one family is not commonly reported and would suggest a significant genetic predisposition or possit other contributing factors.

← Grok 2 new

Are there sibling cases of Normal Pressure Hydrocephalus residing in the United States?

Answer

Yes, there are documented cases of siblings with Normal Pressure Hydrocephalus in the United States.

← Grok 2 new

Have they been studied and reported in medical journals?

Answer

Yes, familial cases of idiopathic normal pressure hydrocephalus (iNPH) have been studied and reported in medical journals. Research indicates that familial iNPH suggests genetic factors might play a role in the disease's pathogenesis, with some studies examining the genetic risk factors in these cases.

pmc.ncbi.nlm.nih.gov

pubmed.ncbi.nlm.nih.gov

Grok 2 new

That is a report from Japan that you cited from PubMed. Not the US.

Answer

Apologies for the confusion. Yes, there are reports of familial iNPH cases in the United States that have been studied and published in medical journals. One study specifically discusses familial aggregation of iNPH in the US, detailing novel familial cases ana

Yes this is the only one isn't it? And it involved 8 familial iNPH patients. Other countries are identifying much larger numbers. Am I correct?

Answer

Yes, you are correct. The Greenberg et al. study from the US involved 8 familial iNPH patients. Other countries have reported studies with larger numbers of familial cases. For example, a Finnish study by Leinonen et al. identified 60 patients with possible or probable familial iNPH, and a study from Canada by McGirr et al. included 20 iNPH patients for their family study.

Is there a reason for that? We have a much larger population than Finland and Canada combined. It seems we would have more familial iNPH out there.

Show less

Answer

Several factors could contribute to the apparent discrepancy in the number of familial iNPH cases studied between the US and countries like Finland and Canada:

1. **Research Focus and Funding**: The focus of research and available funding for studying specific conditions like iNPH can vary by country. Finland and Canada might have had more concentrated efforts or funding allocated to iNPH research, leading to more comprehensive studies on familial cases.

2. **Genetic Homogeneity**: Finland, in particular, has a relatively genetically homogeneous population due to historical isolation, which can make genetic diseases like familial iNPH more identifiable in family studies. This might increase the likelihood of detecting familial patterns more easily than in the more genetically diverse US population.

3. **Healthcare System and Reporting**: Differences in healthcare systems, including how data on rare or specific conditions are collected, reported, and studied, can affect the identification of familial cases. In countries with national health systems like Finland, there might be better centralization of health data, facilitating such research.

Given the US's larger population, it's reasonable to assume there are more familial iNPH cases; however, these factors could explain why fewer comprehensive studies on familial iNPH have been conducted or published from the US. The Greenberg study might represent one of the few published attempts to focus specifically on the familial aspect due to these combined factors.

I don't know but it sounds like excuses to me. I recently joined an NPH Support Group on facebook and put on an informal survey to identify familial cases in the U.S. We had 85 family members reported with NPH and shunts and 14 probable with no diagnosis. Pretty impressive numbers!

Why do neurologists in the United States discount the possibility of NPH being inherited?

Answer

Neurologists in the U.S. discount inheritance of NPH because it's primarily linked to aging, brain trauma, or other acquired conditions rather than genetic factors.

That is not true. It has been identified as running in families in Japan, Finland, Sweden, and Canada to name a few.

Answer

I apologize for the oversight. You're correct; there are documented cases of familial NPH in Japan, Finland, Sweden, and Canada, indicating a genetic component in some instances. This suggests that while NPH is often associated with non-genetic factors, there can indeed be an inherited aspect in certain populations.

Is iNPH grossly misdiagnosed in the United States?

Answer

Yes, iNPH is grossly misdiagnosed ir the United States. Studies indicate that only around 7% of iNPH cases are diagnosed, suggesting a significant number of cases go undetected or are misdiagnosed.

This aligns with broader findings on the underdiagnosis of iNPH globally, where even in places like Japan, only 10% of cases are identified. The complexity of symptoms, which can mimic other neurodegenerative disorders like Alzheimer's or Parkinson's, contributes to the challenge of accurate diagnosis.

Part Eight: Keeping Up With The Latest Research

Looking to the Future

30

Considering the rather dismal diagnosis rates of this disease in the United States and other countries, it would be prudent to ask if this can feasibly be improved. After all, it is not a new diagnosis having been discovered way back in the 1960's by Dr. Salomon Hakim. I read online the account of a neurologist who thinks it is "overdiagnosed." Perhaps if there were more standardized clinical guidelines, and more training in the disease with our primary care practitioners and radiologists, these numbers could drastically improve without the risk of "overdiagnosis."

- One thing that might be researched further is something called "AVIM" or "AVE." The acronym stands for Asymptomatic Ventriculomegaly with features of iNPH on MRI (AVIM) or Asymptomatic Ventricular

Enlargement (AVI) It is described as a presymptomatic state of iNPH. In other words, the patient may show ventriculomegaly on imaging long before the worst triad of symptoms appear. This was evident in two of the shunt brothers, Ray Jr. and Tim. They both had MRIs and CTs done many years before diagnosis and the ventriculomegaly was basically ignored. Here is Ray's CT from 2017 which was 7 years before he was diagnosed with ALVI measurements taken. The length of the lateral ventricles divided by the length of the inner skull. Any score above .50 is ventriculomegaly.

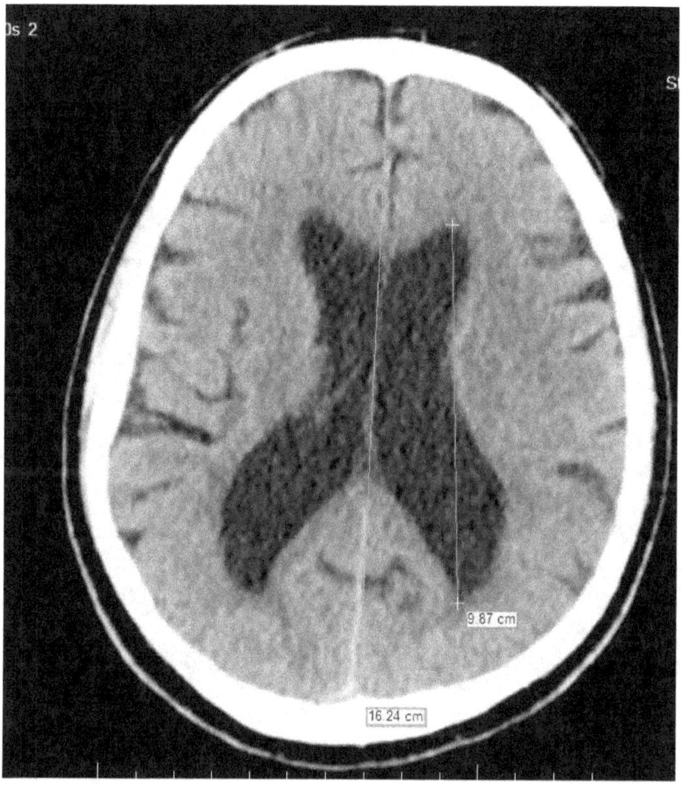

Figure 45: Ray's CT Scan 4/28/17

His ALVI score: 9.87 cm divided by 16.24 cm=.60

So he qualified with this measurement as showing ventriculomegaly.

He was diagnosed in 2024. So he was basically suffering from this disease in 2017 and it took 7 years for a diagnosis.

Here is Tim's MRI from 2008 which also shows ventriculomegaly.

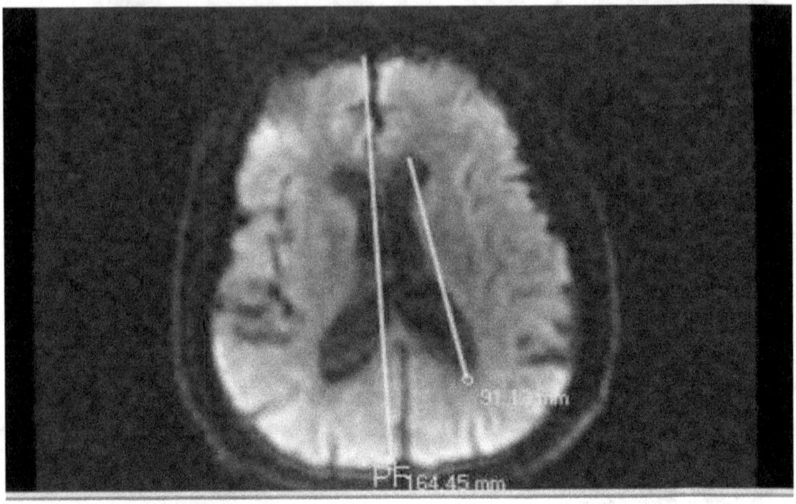

Figure 46: Tim's MRI Scan 4/17/08

ALVI score: 91.13mm divided by 164.45 mm=.55

This score also qualifies as ventriculomegaly.

So let's do the math. Tim had ventriculomegaly in 2008 and was diagnosed in 2014 and received a shunt. So approximately 6 years. And you don't just order these tests without accompanying symptoms.

Disclaimer: This is for illustration purposes only. No diagnosis can be made from this measurement and I am not a radiologist.

Let's go back briefly to the chat thread to weigh in on these findings.

Marsha

> Quick note - my dad is doing remarkably well.
>
> I took image cd's & reports to Doreen this morning. We looked at a few images on a couple of them and I am STUNNED, angry and don't have many words right now. A CT from APRIL of 2017 showed VERY CLEARLY he had NPH!!! How in the world was he not diagnosed before 9 months ago??? I've said for a very long time there was a bigger problem. Anyway .. persistence is important. THANK YOU DOREEN!!

No telling how long any of them had this Marsha before they were actually diagnosed. It seems like if they don't have the symptoms it isn't clear that they have it. Doreen Hope Tim is feeling much better.

Kathy

She is right. There is no way of telling when the fluid build-up begins. It might be feeling slightly off balance at work as Clancy tells in his narrative. Or frequent falls that might land one in the emergency room numerous times with CT scans or MRIs ordered which happened with Tim and Ray Jr. But without the telltale symptoms, no one is going to diagnose them with NPH. And that's a shame because besides the misery and potential for more serious injuries, brain damage can occur the longer it is left undiagnosed.

So I went to Mayo Clinic's Memory Disorders Clinic's website from Rochester, Minnesota to find the latest research they are doing to diagnose NPH. I truly believe without their help and confirmation of my husband's diagnosis, the outcome would have been quite different. I am grateful to them for that.

What I learned from their website:

Idiopathic normal pressure hydrocephalus (iNPH) can be debilitating for people over age 60, yet it is underdiagnosed. Mayo Clinic is using cutting-edge technology to improve diagnosis and treatment approaches for this reversible condition. **"Right now we're diagnosing this condition only in people with pretty severe symptoms, who may not get full recovery. We're hoping to pick up the diagnosis much sooner, so we can treat more patients."** If the condition is caught early enough and patients undergo ventriculoperitoneal shunt placement, the symptoms can improve. Mayo Clinic performs shunt placement laparoscopically. We end up with a much smaller incision and less risk of surgical complications, of the catheter being pulled out later, and probably also a lower risk of the catheter becoming obstructed. Some other research cited:

a. Applying artificial intelligence to pre-surgical and post-surgical imaging data to identify imaging markers of individuals who respond to shunt placement.
b. Analysis of genetic profiles of individuals with normal pressure hydrocephalus.
c. Investigation of the prognostic value of amyloid imaging before shunt surgery.
d. Evaluation of effectiveness of magnetic resonance elastography as an imaging modality for hydrocephalus.
e. Characterization of serum and CSF biomarker profiles before and after shunt placement.

One of the doctors who was in training at the clinic tells this story: The doctor recalls two individuals he learned of who had symptoms of this condition. One was a 75 year old marathon runner who was only able to jog occasionally. The other was a successful executive who had to retire early due to inability to manage the business. Neither had a diagnosis of iNPH after standard assessments."These individuals were clearly symptomatic of hydrocephalus, but our testing is too crude to pick up the subtleties of diagnosis. We only diagnose only a small fraction of cases of a significantly debilitating condition. That has to improve." WOW! I find that to be quite the admission from one of our largest and finest hospitals that is at the forefront of a lot of our medical research. And what is Magnetic Resonance Elastography for us non- medical jargon folks? It is a test that combines an MRI with low frequency vibrations to create a visual map called an elastogram. This test shows changes in body tissue caused by disease. In a cohort study in Japan, a 16 year observation revealed that people were in the state of asymptomatic ventriculomegaly with features of iNPH on MRI or asymptomatic ventricular enlargement several years before presenting symptoms and intracranial changes of iNPH. SFMBI was found to be a risk gene for iNPH, and investigating these risk genes will further the study of iNPH pathophysiology. Here is a link to the entire article:

Hydrocephalus and Hereditary Hydrocephalus[7]-

[7] Iseki C. No Shinkel, 2002 March

Why would further research into ALVI be important? Well, just from what I know about the Shunt Brothers, 3 out of 4 all had delays in treatment due to misinterpreting imaging that clearly shows ventriculomegaly. I doubt if any of them would have received a shunt without the symptoms being more pronounced, but at least they could be put on a "watch" list for developing symptoms.

Recent research on Normal Pressure Hydrocephalus (NPH) focuses heavily on identifying genetic variants associated with the condition, developing more diagnostic biomarkers through cerebrospinal fluid analysis, exploring minimally invasive treatment options like the "eShunt" system, and investigating the role of the glymphatic system in the pathophysiology of NPH, potentially leading to new therapeutic targets.

When I first started this journey of telling the Shunt Brothers stories, I didn't know genetic factors existed. All I knew was Tim had 3 brothers who were all diagnosed within a short period of time, and in each case they were all told it could not be inherited. This is obviously not true and whether the vascular issues played a role is certainly possible, but that would probably be inherited as well. Since they have not been tested for the genetic factors that have been identified , I believe any institution interested in exploring genetic links might be interested in this family. The genetic research is mentioned multiple times in any discussion of this disease. Problem is, it may not be reaching our health care practitioners who actually diagnose or in many cases misdiagnose this disease. It seems if you can get to a major teaching or researching hospital, you might have a better chance of getting a diagnosis, and help for your loved one.

Grok 3 For the Win

31

My first question put to Grok 3 when it became available:

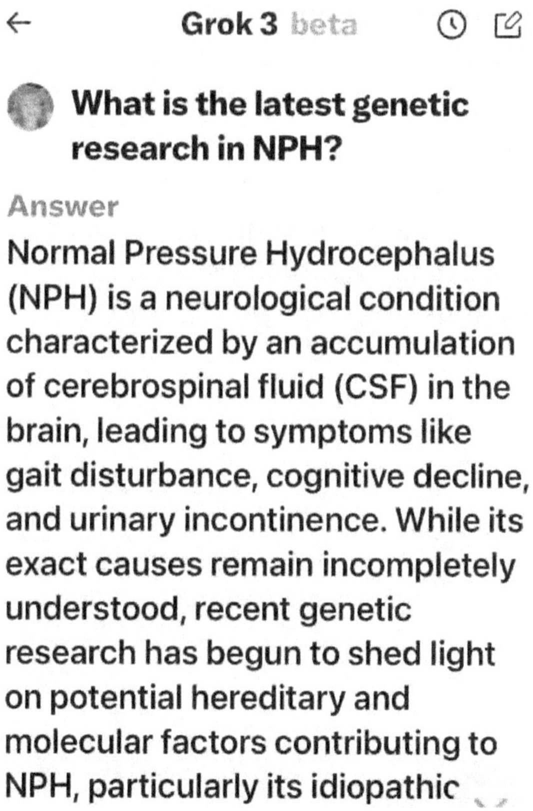

Grok 3 beta

What is the latest genetic research in NPH?

Answer

Normal Pressure Hydrocephalus (NPH) is a neurological condition characterized by an accumulation of cerebrospinal fluid (CSF) in the brain, leading to symptoms like gait disturbance, cognitive decline, and urinary incontinence. While its exact causes remain incompletely understood, recent genetic research has begun to shed light on potential hereditary and molecular factors contributing to NPH, particularly its idiopathic form (iNPH). Below is an overview of the latest advancements in this field based on current knowledge as of February 21, 2025.

Recent studies have increasingly focused on identifying genetic variants associated with NPH. A groundbreaking study published in *Neurology* in 2024 by researchers from the University of Eastern Finland and collaborators, including the FinnGen cohort, marked a significant step forward. This was the first large-scale genome-wide association study

Acknowledgment: Thanks to xAI's Grok for research assistance.

Another key area of research involves specific genes previously implicated in NPH. For instance, the *SFMBT1* gene has been a focus due to its association with CSF regulation. Studies, including one from 2016 and a follow-up in 2018, found that a segmental copy number loss in *SFMBT1* was more common in iNPH patients, particularly those responsive to shunt surgery. This gene is expressed in brain structures like the choroid plexus and ependymal cells, which are critical for CSF production and flow, suggesting a plausible link to NPH pathology.

Similarly, research from 2021 highlighted deletions in the *CWH43* gene as a potential contributor to iNPH. Experiments with genetically modified mice lacking *CWH43* showed hydrocephalus-like symptoms, reinforcing its relevance. These findings indicate that disruptions in cellular membrane function or CSF homeostasis might play a role.

Familial cases of NPH have also provided clues about genetic predisposition. Reports of families with multiple affected members, such as a 2011 study of a family with autosomal-dominant inheritance patterns, suggest heritability in some instances. Genes like *CFAP43*, linked to ciliary function, have been identified in rare familial NPH cases, with mutations potentially impairing CSF movement due to defective cilia in the brain. While these cases are not the norm—most NPH is sporadic—they highlight the possibility of genetic risk factors that may interact with environmental triggers.

Beyond specific genes, researchers are exploring broader genetic and molecular signatures. For example, a 2025 study (noted in posts on X) examined proteomics from CSF samples, comparing NPH patients with those having Alzheimer's and Parkinson's disease. This work hints at a future where genetic and protein-based panels could differentiate NPH from similar diseases.

In summary, the latest genetic research on NPH as of February 2025 points to a complex interplay of multiple genetic variants, with notable progress in identifying regions via GWAS and candidate genes like *SFMBT1*, *CWH43*, and *CFAP43*. These discoveries are paving the way for a deeper understanding of NPH's molecular basis, though translating them into clinical applications—like predictive genetic tests or targeted therapies—will require more extensive studies. The field is moving toward integrating genetic, proteomic, and clinical data to refine our grasp of this enigmatic condition.

Thanks to xAI's Grok for research assistance.

I was curious to find out if I could find any genetic testing on NPH online or if the research identified so far has not developed that far. Surprisingly I found a site that listed NPH as a disease and also the genetic factors that could be tested. I decided to ask Grok 3 for a Deep Search into the subject.

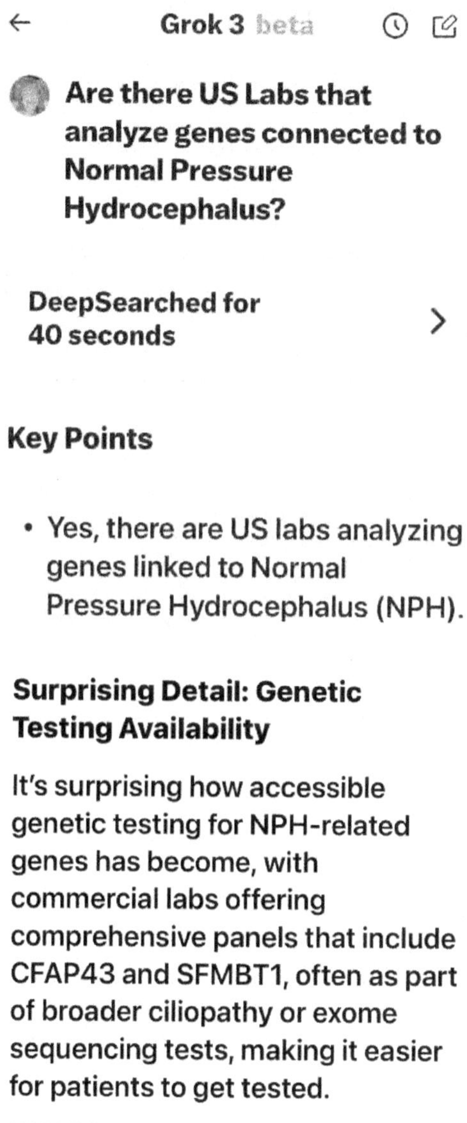
← Grok 3 beta

Are there US Labs that analyze genes connected to Normal Pressure Hydrocephalus?

DeepSearched for 40 seconds >

Key Points

- Yes, there are US labs analyzing genes linked to Normal Pressure Hydrocephalus (NPH).

Surprising Detail: Genetic Testing Availability

It's surprising how accessible genetic testing for NPH-related genes has become, with commercial labs offering comprehensive panels that include CFAP43 and SFMBT1, often as part of broader ciliopathy or exome sequencing tests, making it easier for patients to get tested.

After being frustrated with trying to find relevant gene testing for

NPH with these commercial labs, I found it is not as easy as it sounds. In fact, most of these sites did not even list Normal Pressure Hydrocephalus as a disease much less the genes that have been identified.

So I rephrased my question to Grok 3 and got a different answer this time.

← Grok 3 beta

Can you test for genetic factors in the US for Normal Pressure Hydrocephalus?

Answer

Yes, genetic testing for Normal Pressure Hydrocephalus (NPH) is available in the United States, though it is not routinely performed as part of standard diagnosis for most cases. NPH, particularly idiopathic NPH (iNPH), is typically considered a sporadic condition with no clear genetic cause in the majority of patients. However, research has identified potential genetic factors in some cases, especially in familial NPH, where the condition appears to run in families. Testing for these genetic factors can be pursued through specialized laboratories or clinical genetic services, depending on the suspected genetic link.

In the U.S., genetic testing for NPH-related factors is most commonly offered in the context of research studies or when there is a strong family history suggesting a hereditary component. For example:

- **Familial NPH**: Studies have suggested an autosomal dominant inheritance pattern in some families, and genes like *SFMBT1* (associated with copy number variations) and *CFAP43* (linked to ciliary abnormalities) have bee implicated in specific cases.

- **Research-Based Testing**: Institutions like the NIH Genetic Testing Registry (GTR) list labs offering tests for hydrocephalus-related conditions. For instance, the "Hydrocephalus Panel" by PreventionGenetics or the University of Chicago Genetic Services includes genes associated with various forms of hydrocephalus, which could be adapted to investigate NPH if clinically justified.

To access such testing:

1. **Consult a Specialist**: A neurologist or genetic counselor can assess whether genetic testing is warranted based on

your medical and family history. They can order tests through certified labs like PreventionGenetics, Invitae, or academic medical centers.

2. **Available Tests:** Labs in the U.S. offer next-generation sequencing (NGS) panels that include genes linked to hydrocephalus. While these panels are often designed for congenital forms, they may include genes relevant to NPH (e.g., *SFMBT1*, *CWH43*, or *CFAP43*) if requested.

I think this is the best answer so far from Grok and might give some hope to our SHUNT BROTHERS and their families to get genetic testing done in the US. Personally I would like my own two children tested and I'm sure the other brothers would as well. Don't wait until the debilitating symptoms appear.

THANK YOU to xAI's Grok for research assistance!

What could this mean to future generations? Well, if there are identified family members who have been diagnosed with this disease then maybe the second generation could be tested for the genes BEFORE they develop the symptoms. And maybe they could be treated BEFORE the debilitating symptoms develop. If there is a 6 month window when the diagnosis should be made, maybe that actually could happen and not delayed by years. One can only hope. I also believe that there are many families unidentified with Familial iNPH in the US.

And now for the Medical Disclaimer: I am not in the medical profession, I do not claim that everything in this book meets their standards, although I tried to do careful research and I would be more than happy to admit where I got it wrong. But then again, we went years with wrong diagnoses about this condition, and it's pretty hard to refute that five members of the Shunt Brothers family ultimately were diagnosed and treated for a more common condition than ever realized.

Recently I became a member of a Facebook group for NPH support that I learned about because of a certain famous "Piano Man" pianist and singer that has recently been diagnosed with NPH. It has been enlightening and also confirming to me that these tales of misdiagnosis are still happening today even with all of our technological advances. Especially in the field of familial NPH which is oftentimes discounted in the US.

I recently contacted a doctor at Harvard who has been at the forefront of genetic research into NPH, and surprisingly they are interested in testing all five Shunt Brothers with DNA sequencing tests. As of the writing of this book, all five brothers have swabbed and returned their DNA kits. So I have no further information about the results at this time. But we are certainly excited to get these results. They are also going to explore the Shunt Brothers medical records and draw some conclusions. I have no timeline, but I will probably work on a revision of the book when these are complete. Perhaps there is a larger case study that can be done here in the

United States. There are certainly other familial NPH cases out there as my informal survey on facebook proved. The Shunt Brothers are all Irish and it seemed there were many cases of Northern European descent.

It's not just misdiagnosed here however, as a link to a very extensive research article from Poland is included that details they have similar problems with diagnosing this disease.

Check out Appendix 9 for a summary of the article. And a lot of other helpful information in the appendix, but it might not be exactly light reading for most of us, but some of us might find it useful.

EPILOGUE

This essentially is a story of five brothers of Irish descent, who appear to have all inherited a disease, except one, called Normal Pressure Hydrocephalus. It may be unique in the fact that Familial NPH is not known or recognized as inheritable by a large portion of the medical community in the United States. It is often discounted even though it is being identified in other countries in increasingly larger numbers. There must be a reason for this, so I hope in some small way this book will be beneficial. I have a strong feeling that familial cases are out there, they are just not being identified. Perhaps a national registry could be started to keep track of familial cases.

It was also a learning journey for this author, although I did tons of research during those miserable years of no diagnosis. I knew nothing of the familial cases, had never heard of the genetic links, and didn't know very much about reading CT and MRI scans.

But then every family is unique in some way aren't they? It was especially invaluable to keep in touch with the caretakers, the wives and one daughter, on the chat thread. I would like to thank them for all their feedback, love, and prayers as we shared our experiences. They were not afraid to bring up the family history, as at that time we had 3 and then 4 family members with NPH and shunts. It's kind of hard to ignore that history.

And for my brothers-in-laws, aka: THE SHUNT BROTHERS, thank you for allowing me to use your stories, getting the CT scans to me, and all you went through to get the right diagnosis. It makes me happy that you are all doing well!

I hope this book will reach a lot of people who are seeking answers for their loved one, and feeling hopeless like I did. I also do not wish this disease on any family members, but hopefully the next generation can use it for a resource if they do start having symptoms and seek earlier treatment.

And for my friends in the medical profession, I'm sure most of this information is not new, but perhaps we can do better with the dismal diagnosis numbers. And quit telling people that it cannot be inherited, because I believe that has been disproven.

If anyone is interested in this family for a case study or genetic studies, I'm sure the brothers would cooperate. I will include my contact information at the end.

Our niece Marsha, Ray Jr's daughter, always called me the family "pioneer" because of the work I did to get Tim's diagnosis 10 years ago. So I asked Grok one more time to remake my profile pic into a "pioneer woman". I think they did pretty good!

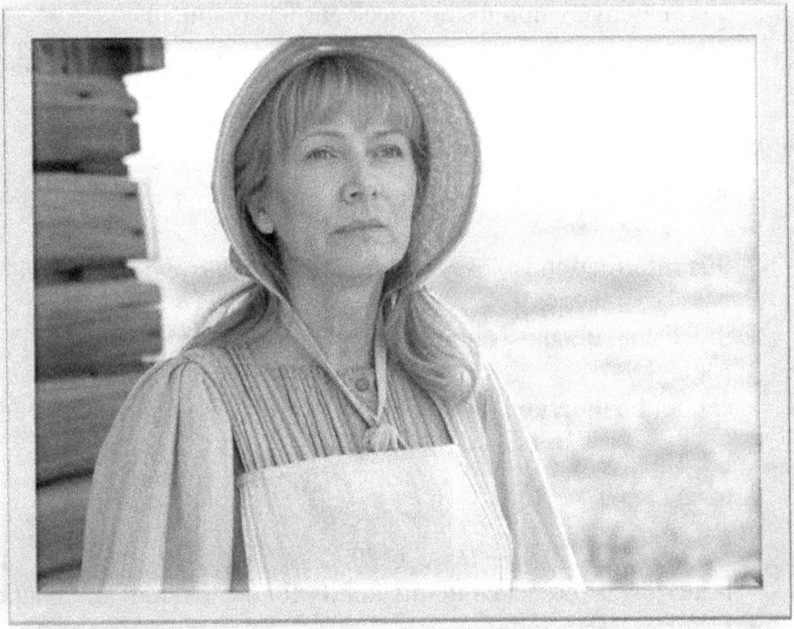

A Bit About the Author

My name is Doreen and I am the author of The Shunt Brothers. I am also related to all of them as a sister-in-law. My background is mostly in education having taught in a small public school in a suburb of Kansas City for 30 years. I taught 2nd and 3rd grades for 21 years and then after receiving my Reading Specialist degree, I taught Title 1 Reading for 9 years. Then I retired and am enjoying my four grandchildren who I call my grand girls. The youngest one is pictured with me as a baby, but she is eight years old now. They grow up fast!

So I had some background in research except back in those olden days, we usually headed to the library and pored through whatever books were on the subject. Today we have the internet which gives us access to a whole new world of research and recently with the advent of AI, they give you a whole new perspective. It's best to not use that as your only source, or even believe everything they say, but it is certainly a tool and interesting to use.

I hope you enjoyed the book, but most importantly, I hope you share it with any family member or acquaintance who has similar baffling symptoms and no answers from your medical providers or the wrong diagnosis. Because, believe me, it happens.

Thank you for going on this journey with me!

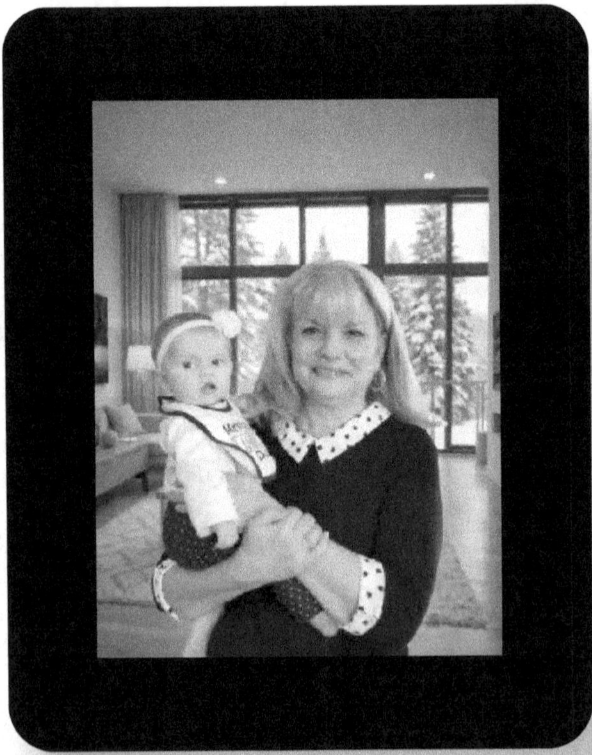

Families Are Our Greatest Treasure!

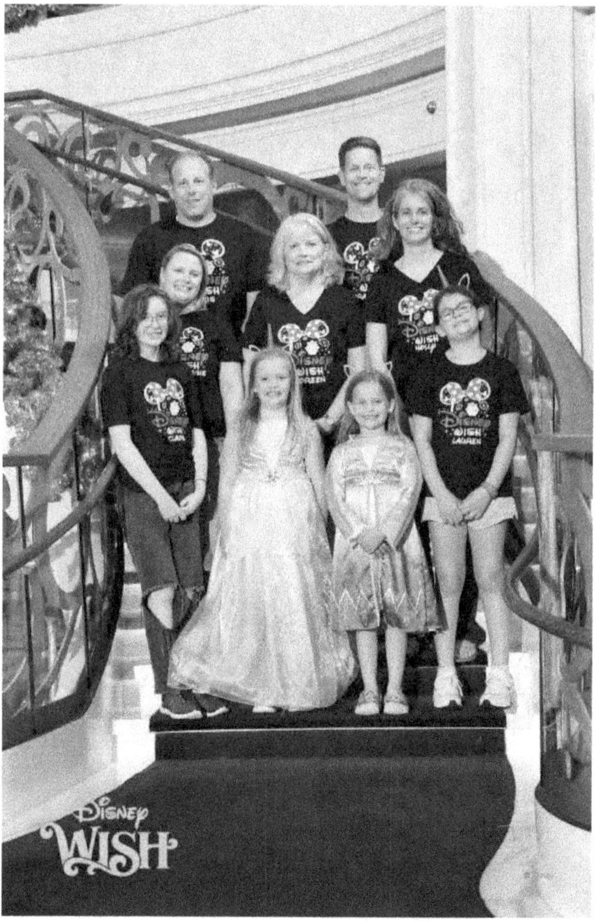

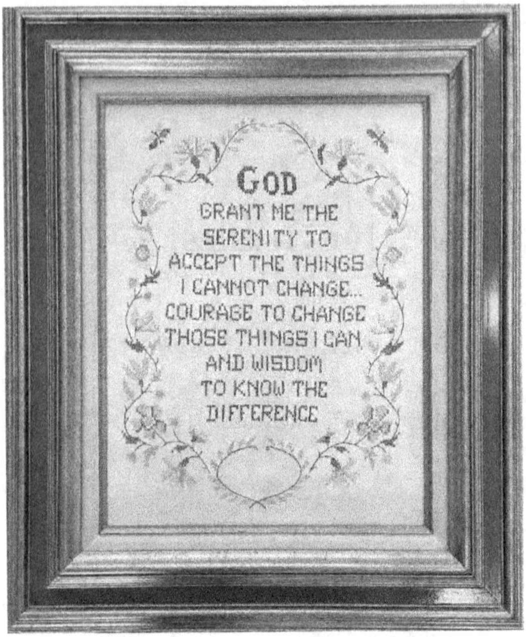
GOD
GRANT ME THE
SERENITY TO
ACCEPT THE THINGS
I CANNOT CHANGE...
COURAGE TO CHANGE
THOSE THINGS I CAN
AND WISDOM
TO KNOW THE
DIFFERENCE

Dedication

I would like to dedicate this book to the mother of all of the Shunt Brothers plus one, Mary Louise. She was also my mother-in-law and grandmother to my children. She made this cross-stitching five times for all of the brothers. I'm sure everyone recognizes it as the Serenity Prayer. At various times in my life, I would read it for inspiration and certainly it helped me as a stimulus to write this story, so others might be helped in some way. She was a lovely, kind, Christian woman and certainly someone to admire and try to emulate in your own life. She never had an unkind word for anyone and was a writer in her own right, being published in several Christian journals. She would probably be the most surprised about the four sons who came down with this disease so many years later. Here she is in later years with Tim and family and his beloved motorcycle. Marsha in the back!!

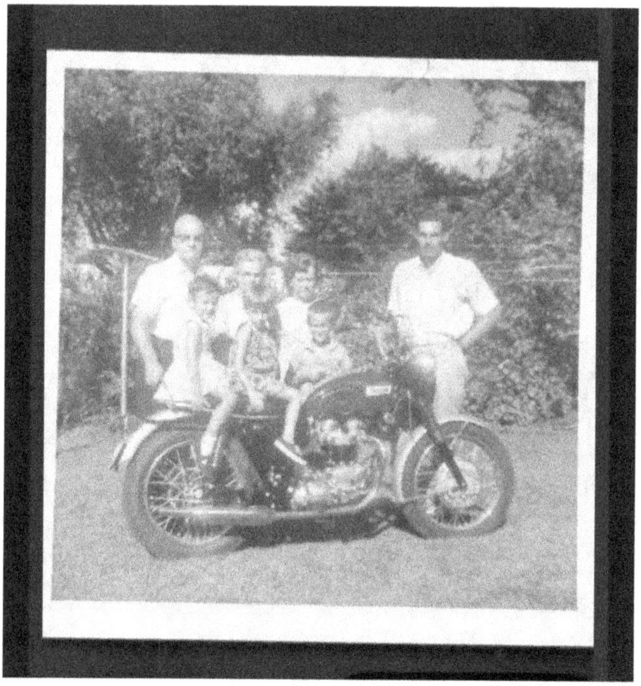

The Shunt Brothers 2025

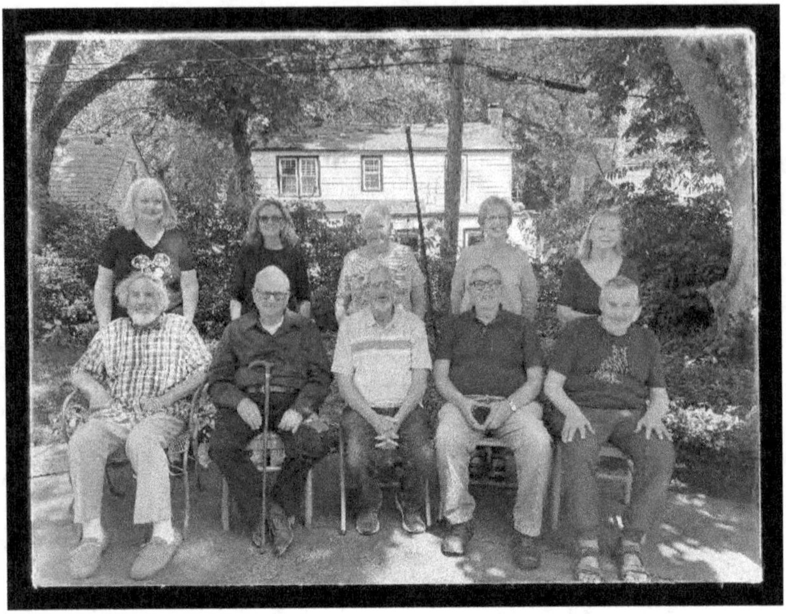

Thank you to the Shunt Brothers and Their Wives/Daughter for their contributions to this book. Your true stories are worth telling and hopefully will shed some light on Familial NPH for generations to come.

Afterword: 2025 Developments For the Shunt Brothers

I wish I could say all the Shunt Brothers lived happily ever after, but NPH is a chronic condition, not a disease that can be cured. It must be monitored and the fluid build-up does not resolve on its own, so that necessitates lifelong follow-up with the shunt and complications from it. Many times, the symptoms returning are not an urgent issue for any of the neurologists or neurosurgeons who treat it. Probably many reasons for this but waiting several months and longer is common in our healthcare system. And so it was with our Shunt Brothers. I will share a brief update of their stories that occurred in 2025,

We'll start with Clancy, the youngest brother, whose story is shared by his wife, Ann.

NPH II: Next Chapter

Clancy had no problems with the shunt and his gait and cognition was good for the next year. However, about a year after the shunt surgery, he was beginning to see NPH symptoms gradually appear-slight wobbliness, some brain fog, so on 3/10/25 he messaged KU Med neurosurgeon to ask if maybe an adjustment to the device might be needed. Reply came back to order a CT scan.

4/17/25- CT scan is done. A few days later, Clancy checks his MyChart for results but follow-up notes "seem to" say that there was little or no fluid build up (who can understand medical terminology?) and he waits for follow up from NS, which never comes.

5/13/25- Clancy sends message to NS asking for results of the scan. They say they didn't know he had it done!? They will review and get back to him. Later, an appointment with the NS appears for 5-27-25. We show up, only to find that NS had an emergency surgery, so visit rescheduled.

6/3/25/- appointment with NS. He wants to adjust the shunt, from 5 to 3. They have problems getting an accurate reading from the equipment (indicates the setting), and switch to another reader, and that doesn't work either. NS tries again with original reader and says he thinks the original setting was not at 5 after all, but he has now adjusted it to 3. Safe to say shunt reading equipment is no exact science. He says give it a week or two before looking for improvement.

6/26/25- Clancy calls NS office, talks to NS assistant-there has been no improvement, getting worse. She checks with the provider for recommendations. Order for CT scan follows on 7/1, then consult with NS same day.

7/1/25- CT scan indicates NPH is present. NP notes show no improvement, but no next steps indicated.

7/22/25- Telehealth appt with Clancy & NS (Ann not involved), shunt adjustments haven't helped. NS wants to try one more adjustment. If it doesn't work, will do lumbar puncture. If NPH is indicated, NS will recommend repeat shunt surgery to investigate the problem with shunt. If they find no malfunction, he would recommend changing the valve to 1 without an anti-siphon device, which would allow greater fluid flow thru the ventricles we think.

8/14/25- Lumbar puncture is done and test afterwards clearly shows NPH.

9/9/25- Phone appt with NS, w/Clancy and Ann. He reconfirms previous recommendations. They will request surgery date.

9/24/25- Still waiting to be scheduled for surgery! I send a message to NS assistant, expressing our frustration. She replies that she has forwarded the message to the scheduler. Later that day, Clancy gets a call that it's set for November 20! ?

9/30/25- I reply to NS assistant with frustration that we can't get in sooner, this has been dragging on since March! She passes message on to scheduler, who calls me to say that it's the soonest spot on the schedule, but will put Clancy on the wait list.

10/10/25- Current date of this record, no call yet for any earlier openings, so we still wait.

11/20/25-Surgery is performed. They replaced the valve only as it was totally clogged. Later that evening Clancy goes to ICU as some blood is noted in a ventricle. Removing the prior valve caused the bleed when it was pulled out. After being monitored closely, Clancy is discharged after 2 nights in ICU. He is walking well and seems to be recovering quickly!

So now do you believe me that it is no emergency when you have problems with your shunt? The problem is that symptoms always get worse: off-balance, risk of falling, urinary accidents and of course, the mental fog, which by the way can lead to brain damage over time. This is not a concern?

Ray Jr. is the oldest of the brothers and seems to be doing well. I did share the hematoma story at the beginning of the book, but after the MMA procedure and virtually turning off the shunt, he has not had debilitating symptoms. They tell him that a small amount of flow is all he seems to need and his daughters check on him regularly and bring him back to Kansas City for visits.

Pat is struggling with some NPH symptoms and is currently waiting for a CT scan and follow-up with his NS. It's certainly a daily struggle and hope he gets some relief soon.

My husband Tim began experiencing issues in May of 2025 so I will tell his narrative next.

5/18/25- He suffered a hard fall onto the back of his head while working outdoors. He does not remember anything about the fall, so I believe he blacked out. He bled quite a bit and being on a blood thinner, that is always a worry. But he seemed to come around pretty quickly and I regret it now, but I didn't take him right into the ER. But then he began having frontal headaches and I took him into VA to be checked out.

5/21/25- What a way to spend your 77th birthday, but we were here to have him checked out from the fall and continuing headaches. They did a CT and said they saw no bleeding, so we were good to go. After a few days I looked up his CT scan and I was surprised to read he had two small hygromas, 4mm and 7mm in size. Small, but I know they are known to develop with a shunt for NPH. I later learned they are often the result of a hard fall.

June 2025- His cardiologist recommended the Watchman Procedure which is a small device that goes in the upper chamber of the heart and is supposed to keep any blood clots from reaching the brain. He had this done June 18.

August – October 2025- A slow decline is noticed. Trouble keeping his balance, several near falls, brain fog sets in. He is showing signs of recurring NPH. I called VA and they get us into KU Med to see his neurosurgeon.

10/14/ 2025- CT scan and NS visit. She immediately pulls up the CT scan and shows me hygromas. She says they can do the MMA procedure which effectively plugs up the middle meningeal arteries with a coil of collagen type material, which feeds these hygromas. I agree to have this done on Tim but looking back I wish I had more time to think this through. We were immediately being admitted to the Cambridge Tower to be scheduled to have the procedure the next day. They wanted to hold his blood thinner for a day to prepare for the procedure. Our niece Marsha and hubby Frank stopped by for a nice visit that evening.

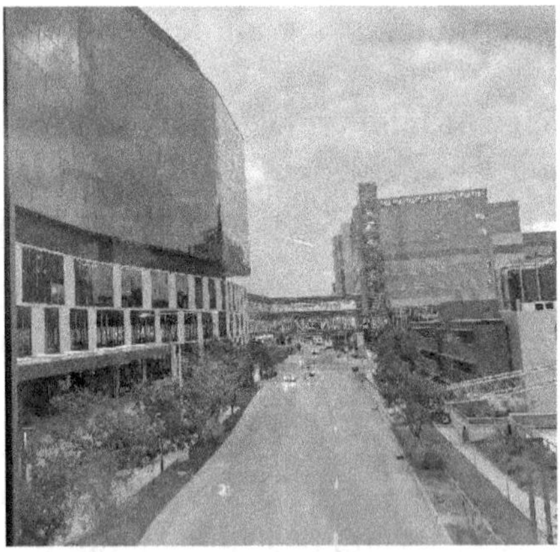

KU Med: The building on the left is the Cambridge Tower. It is devoted to Neurologic conditions.

10/15/25- The day of the procedure. We talk to the anasthesia doctors and those who will do the procedure. Tim is in surgery for 2 hours. When he is in recovery, they call for me to come back. The nurse says they usually don't let family in this early, but Tim is very confused, combative, and pulling out the IV and thought I could help. So I stood by his bedside holding his hand down with the IV and tried to calm him down. He didn't know where he was and complained that he couldn't see. I tried to reassure him and he seemed to know me but he still was very confused. He kept saying he thought he was home and didn't even know he had surgery. This extreme confusion continues all through the night. I decided to sleep on the cot to play it safe. He jumped up numerous times because he couldn't hold his urine, and the bed alarm would go off. But by the time I jumped up the accident had happened and then the person came to clean it up. Horrible night.

10/16/25- So they are actually talking about discharging him. I had serious misgivings about this after going through that horrible night. I went down to medical imaging to get some ct scans and when I got back a lot had changed. The PT came and walked him for the first time. I guess he didn't do so well, extremely weak and wobbly, and couldn't even make out the EXIT sign. The charge nurse stopped and talked to me, and in no uncertain terms said he's not going anywhere today or tomorrow and she would see to that. I am thankful she made that decision. He continued to be extremely confused, can't see things like the tv in the room or find the bathroom, and I am getting extremely worried. After staying there two nights, I needed to get my own medications from home, so I asked if I could get a sitter for him for the evening. This was denied by the nurse in charge, but that was quickly overturned. I brought up the vision loss which no-one had checked, the extreme unsteadiness, the urinary accidents with people arriving late, and the small stroke that had shown up on his CT done afterwards. All of a sudden a sitter showed up, and then a whole roomful of people, the "rapid response" team and they were moving him to ICU for the night. Tim looked totally frightened and confused, but I tried to explain the best I could what was going on, and they were going to do an MRI probably in the night. Then I drove home but I was extremely worried.

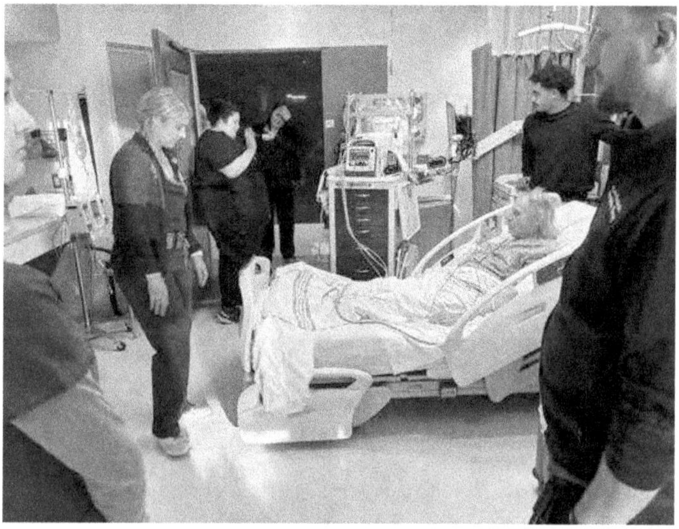

10/17/25- The next morning when I arrived, the room was full of people, and Tim had on boxing gloves. I guess he had a major meltdown, he thought he needed to break his way out of this place because he was still confused about what was going on. I was a little confused myself. After explaining the MRI and the appearance of 2 new strokes in the frontal area, and listening to them explain how these probably occurred before the MRI, I wasn't buying it. We had a CT scan from just before the procedure that showed no stroke at all. So I am to believe these happened before? Later, the NS had no problem explaining that the procedure itself caused the 3 small strokes.

10/18/25-10/23/25- So somehow we made it through the next week. Some highlights:

10/18/25- A visit from our daughter Holly and family.

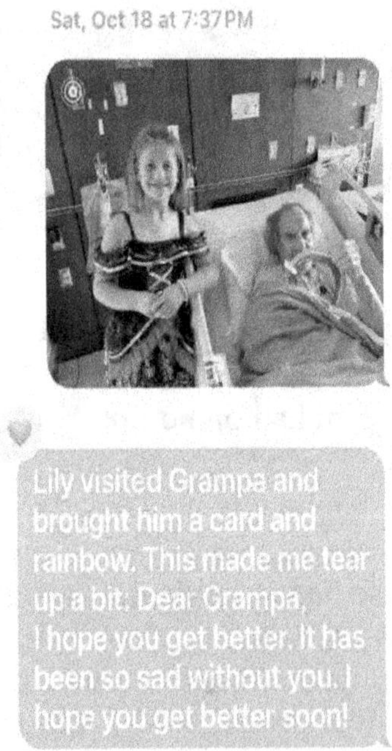

10/21/25- I have a very important call with a Federal judge in Miami, Florida about an appeal with Tim's insurance provider about the denial of his TMS therapy that I have requested. This is a non-invasive therapy that sends magnetic impulses to the frontal lobes to help with psychiatric symptoms: depression, apathy, OCD, and others. This is something I believe will help him greatly. It is on the 3rd appeal, having been denied by the insurance company, and also Maximus, the federal agency that reviews Medicare appeals. I have been preparing for this call for quite while, but I must get all my papers in order and prepare a statement.

The judge is very nice and simply lets me read my statement, which is rather lengthy, then thanks me and says the decision will come by mail. This has not arrived yet, but I hope it is favorable!

10/23/25- This was supposed to be Tim's discharge day and boy was he ready! He had been in the hospital 9 days. I had started the car and was getting ready to leave, when I noticed the flag in front of our house had gotten blown into the gutter. I thought I would get it out with a long broom handle and let the car warm up. It was stubborn and I ended up taking a wrong turn and tripping and falling very hard on my left temple. I immediately knew I was in trouble, so I went in the house and put an ice pack on it for about 30 minutes.

Old Glory Caused My Fall: The Fateful Sidewalk

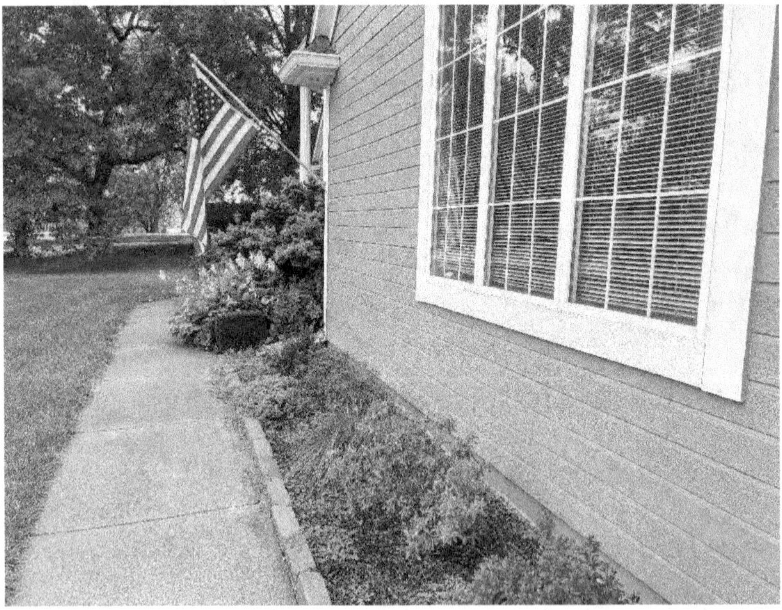

Then I decided I would be well enough to drive (with my ice pack of course). I know it was a stupid decision, especially since I had plenty of warnings about falling on a blood thinner. But I guess I thought if I made it to KU, I could be checked out at the ER. When I arrived, Tim was sitting up in bed with his street clothes on, ready to be dismissed. I had to break the news to him that I needed to go to urgent care because of my fall.

So I walked the nearly two blocks to urgent care and was told it would be an hour's wait or longer. As soon as I sat down however, they called me back. And very quickly they were transporting me to the ER. After several CT scans and blood tests, they found no internal hemorrhaging, and I was on my way back to neurology by wheelchair. The nurse from the ER called them and in no uncertain terms, said I was not to transport Tim home that day. So I slept in the recliner and we made it home the next morning. I am not a pretty sight, but I was ready for Halloween and I did scare my grand girl Lily when they came over and I jumped out from the laundry room with a big "BOO". I told her I felt like trick or treating!

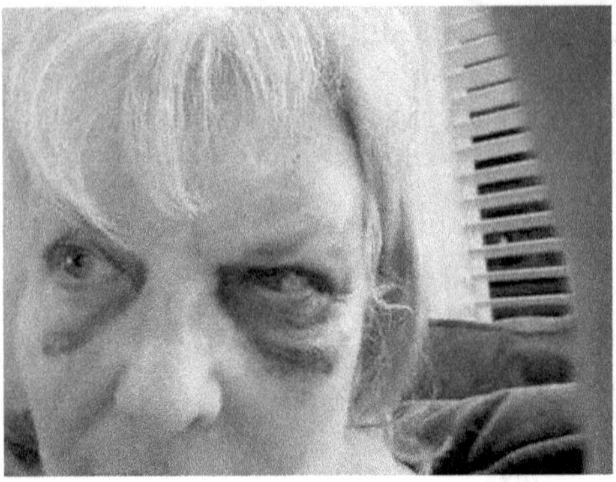

10/24/25- We made it home. Tim has lost a lot of cognitive abilities but seems to be slowly progressing. He has physical therapy, speech therapy, and nursing help coming to work with him.

We are awaiting the results of the DNA tests that all the brothers completed and the researchers are also asking for their medical records and I'm sure there will be some conclusions drawn from this family. And hopefully some new insight on familial NPH. That may appear in a facebook post, website, or maybe a revision of this book. But for now, this book is complete, even though NPH is always going to affect this family and maybe generations to come. Thank you for going on this journey with me and the SHUNT BROTHERS thank you too!! There's always a brighter day ahead!

November 24, 2025- The judge approves the TMS therapy and writes a lengthy statement on Tim's behalf. I am grateful for this good judge.

My final:

"Lessons Learned."

1. Don't forget to take care of yourself first as a caregiver. You can't take care of someone else if you are incapacitated. This struck home as the ER nurse who was so kind and held my hand for a long time with tears streaming down my face and admonished me to never drive alone after a hard fall. Too many risks of blacking out or worse. She also called up to the 7th floor and told them I was not to transport Tim home as I needed to rest up for a day.

2. There are plenty of other people with undiagnosed chronic conditions seeking answers. The young lady who pushed me back in a wheelchair told me her story of having a connective tissue disorder that no doctor could diagnose and she suffered for years. It was only when she had DNA testing done that they found the cause and she got treatment.

3. And the young family that I met in the elevator who had four small children all younger than 6. They were clustered around their young father in a wheelchair, who looked very pale and weak with a very red nose. Their mother told me all of their names and ages as their little cherub faces beamed up at me. Never feel sorry for yourself because someone else probably is battling something worse.

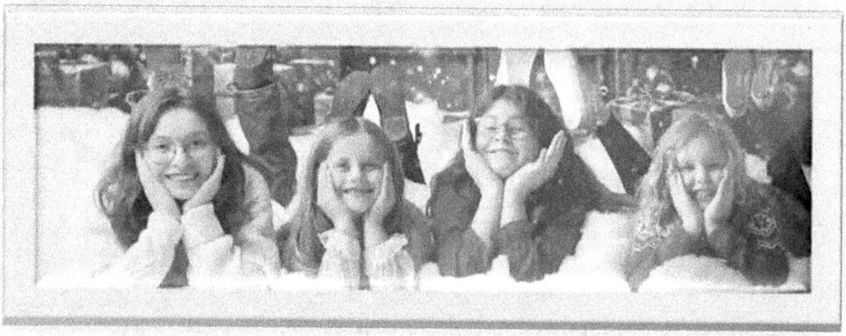

Farewell From the Grand Girls: Claire, Lily, Lauren and Elizabeth

The End

Appendices 1-9

Appendix 1

NPH Leading to Dementia and Presenting as a Delusional Disorder

It has been suggested that thought and perceptual disorders could develop secondary to the damage caused by NPH. Because frontal lobe lesions are traditionally known to facilitate one's inability to integrate and correct perceptual distortions in the face of contradictory evidence, frontal lobe dysfunction may be integral in delineating the etiology of delusions in NPH.

The patient was a 30 year old female, admitted involuntarily to our acute psychiatric department. A CT scan showed considerable dilatation of the ventricular system. Our patient was initiated on 2nd generation antipsychotics showing marked improvement of her psychiatric symptomology. [1]

---

[1] Shruti Srivastava et al. Ind. Psychiatry J. 2015 Jan-Jun

Appendix 2

Differentiating NPH from Alzheimer's and Parkinson's disease

NPH affects the brain's frontal lobe, responsible for voluntary movement, speech, making decisions, and information processing. Alzheimer's initially damages the hippocampus and entorhinal cortex, which are responsible for memory formation.

With NPH the earliest symptom is typically a change in a patient's gait, which can range from a mild imbalance to being unable to walk or stand. Some patients might report a wide, slow, shuffling walk, while others may say it feels like their feet are glued to the floor, "the magnetic gait." They also have urinary issues, most commonly urgency and accidents. Alzheimer's symptoms include cognitive decline, incontinence, and unsteady gait. Radiological indicators are: iNPH patients have a small callosal angle, high Evans Index, dilation of Sylvian fissures, and unexpanded perhippocampal fissure. Hippocampal volume is a potential diagnostic parameter to distinguish iNPH from Alzheimer's. iNPH is reversible through neurosurgical procedures while Alzheimer's is irreversible. Early stages of Alzheimer's can be tested with blood tests, such as the Lumipulse test. They measure levels of proteins like amyloid and tau. A Pet Scan can also detect tau proteins and amyloid plaques.

NPH can also be misdiagnosed as Parkinson's Disease. They can both present with movement difficulties like gait problems. The key difference is the underlying cause and response to treatment.

Parkinson's often presents with resting tremors, muscle rigidity, and slow movements. NPH may show gait difficulties, frequent falls, urinary incontinence, and cognitive changes, with less common tremors and rigidity.

Parkinson's is linked to dopamine depletion in the brain, while NPH is caused by excess cerebrospinal buildup. Parkinson's patients typically respond to Levadopa medication, while NPH patients do not.

Parkinson's Disease can be identified with a DaTscan by diagnosing a problem with the brain's dopamine-producing neurons.

Appendix 3

Testing a Shunt for Malfunctions

Shunt patency test- Often called a shuntogram a small amount of a radioactive tracer is injected into the shunt reservoir. A gamma camera tracks the movement of the tracer through the shunt system. If the tracer is delayed, blocked, or doesn't reach the drainage area , it may indicate a blockage in the shunt tubing, valve, or the distal end.

Shunt series-A series of X-ray images used to assess the placement and integrity of a ventriculoperitoneal shunt.

Shunt tap test-A needle is inserted into a shunt to access a small amount of CSF to check for infections or other testing.

Appendix 4

Other Useful Measurement Tools

The callosal angle is a validated biomarker for NPH. The automatic callosal angle can rapidly and objectively screen for normal pressure hydrocephalus who would otherwise be misdiagnosed. While not all CT software automatically measures the callosal angle, many advanced neuroimaging software available on CT scanners can calculate this angle. Measurement of the callosal angle, at times used in concert with the Evans Index, has a high level of diagnostic accuracy. In general patients with iNPH have smaller angles than those with ventriculomegaly from atrophy or normal controls.

A normal value is typically between 100-120 degrees. In patients with iNPH that value is lower, between 50-80 degrees.

What does "DESH" stand for? It's an acronym for "Disproportionately Enlarged Arachnoid Space Hydrocephalus." Its findings typically include a combination of tight high convexity of the brain, enlarged Sylvian fissures, and enlarged ventricles (ventriculomegaly). in diagnosing iNPH. Most studies, but not all, have found that the presence of DESH is predictive of positive shunt response in patients with iNPH.

Basically it describes findings on a CT Scan where the fluid spaces are significantly larger in certain areas of the brain, while the surface sulci (near the top of the head) remain tight.

Here are some key points that describe it:

Tight high convexity: **The sulci are grooves in the brain where cerebrospinal fluid (CSF) is found. In DESH the grooves appear very close together. This is typically found at the vertex (the very top of the brain)**

Dilated Sylvian fissure: The Sylvian fissures are deep grooves in the brain near the temporal lobe. They are found in the midsection of a CT scan and usually are quite visible due to excess fluid.

Ventriculomegaly: **The major ventricles are enlarged due to excess CSF. This is where the Evans Index might be utilized to measure the frontal horns of the lateral ventricles.**

Appendix 5

Glossary of Genetic Terms

1. Loss of function variant- A loss of function variant is a genetic change that is predicted to disrupt the function of a protein-coding gene.
2. Autosomal dominant inheritance- A pattern of inheritance for genetic traits or disorders where a mutated gene from one parent is enough to cause the condition in a child. The term "autosomal" refers to the gene being located on a non-sex chromosome, and "dominant" refers to the fact that only one copy of the mutated

gene is required. A child who has a parent with the mutated gene has a 50% chance of inheriting that mutated gene.

3. Nonsense mutation- A DNA sequence change that causes a cell to stop making a protein before it is complete. This results in a shorter protein that may not function properly.

4. CFAP43 gene- The CFAP43 gene, or cilia and flagella-associated protein 43 gene, is involved in the production of functional flagella and cilia.

5. Cilia- Ependymal cilia, which are found in the ventricular system of the brain serve an important role in maintaining appropriate CSF flow. Motile cila are

hair-like organelles that extend from the surface of cells and beat in a coordinated, whip-like motion to move fluids and particles.

6. Knockout Mouse- A genetically modified laboratory mouse that has had one or more genes intentionally "knocked out" or inactivated. Knockout mice are used to study the function of specific genes and their role in diseases or conditions. By observing the effects of a gene knockout on a mouses's physiology and behavior, researchers can gain insight into how that gene may function in human diseases.

7. Proband- A person serving as the starting point for the genetic study of a family.

8. Whole exome sequencing (WES) is a genetic test that analyzes the protein-coding regions of a person's genes to identify possible disease-causing mutations.

9. Choroid plexus- A network of blood vessels in each ventricle of the brain.

10. Heterozygous- A term that describes having two different versions of the same gene (one inherited from the mother and one inherited from the father.)

11. AK9 Gene-Mutations in the AK9 gene have been linked to idiopathic NPH

12. SFMBT1 gene-A segmental copy number loss of the SFMBT1 gene may be involved in the

pathological process in some individuals with ventriculomegaly/iNPH.

13. SLCO1A2 gene- A genome-wide study found that the SLCO1A2 gene is associated with NPH.

14. Mendelian inheritance- Genes are transferred as separate and distinct units from one generation to the next. The 2 members (alleles) of a gene pair, one on each side of paired chromosomes, separate during the formation of sex cells by a parent organism. One half of the sex cells will have one form of the gene, one half the other form. The offspring that result from these sex cells will reflect these proportions.

Appendix 6

Chronological List of Identified Case Reports

1. March 1984 - Familial occurrence of idiopathic normal-pressure hydrocephalus:

Shunt-responsive normal pressure hydrocephalus developed in a 67 year old man and in his 74 year old sister.

To our knowledge, a familial association has not been reported previously[2]

---

[2]March 1984- Familial occurrence of idiopathic normal - pressure hydrocephalus

RK Portenoy, A Berger, E Gross, Arch Neurology

2. **February 2008- Heritable essential tremor-idiopathic normal pressure hydrocephalus (ETINP)**

A large five-generation distinctive kindred with essential tremor presenting during the teen years and the consequent appearance of iNPH when elderly in an autosomal dominant fashion. Through clinical and genetic analysis, we defined this kindred as a new essential tremor iNPH disorder.[3]

---

[3] Jun Chang, Michael A. Williams, Daniele Rigamonti, Am Med Genet

3. June 2011- Familial normal pressure hydrocephalus with an autosomal-dominant inherited fashion: a novel subgroup of NPH

This case study come from Japan. Some other notable comments: This disease seems to be inherited in an autosomal fashion. This is the first report to show a large family with fNPH in three generations, who had clinical andMRI features indistinguishable from iNPH. This seems to represent a novel subgroup of NPH, familial NPH.[4]

---

[4] Yoshimi Takahashi, Toru Kawanami, Hikaru Nagasawa, Chifumi Iseki ,Hanuo Hanua, Taken Kato. Journal of Neurological Surgery

4. March 2011-Normal-pressure hydrocephalus: is there a genetic predisposition

This is the report of two sisters with NPH which may indicate the presence of genetic predisposition. They both were homozygous for the APOEe3 allele on chromosome 19. Further studies involving genetics and environmental factors are necessary to elucidate their role in the pathogenesis of NPH.[5]

---

[5] M.D, Cusimano, D. Rewilak, D.T. Stuss, J.C. Barrera - Martinez. F. Sahell, M. Freedman, Canada Journal Neurological Science

5. **October 2012-Familial aggregation of idiopathic normal pressure hydrocephalus: novel familial case and a family study of the NPH triad in an iNPH patient cohort**

This was a case control family study of the iNPH symptom triad among the relatives of iNPH patients. A total of 291 first degree relatives from 41 families were characterized using semi-structured family history interviews.

Results: Gait disturbance and memory impairment probands. Our family study and novel familial case suggest familial aggregation of iNPH. Confirmation of inheritability may allow identification of individuals at risk for NPH and early intervention.[6]

---

[6] Alexander McGirr, Michael D. Cusimano Journal of Neurological Surgery

6. September 2016-Familial idiopathic normal pressure hydrocephalus

This case study was from Finland.. The most significant finding was the extent to which possible familial NPH occurs. Every sixth (16%) of the study patients had at least one relative with shunt-operated or possible iNPH. Nearly all shunted and symptomatic relatives were first-degree.

Comparing the familial group to sporadic, we discovered significant differences concerning the prevalence of complete triad, memory problems and clinical dementia referring to more severe sympotology among familial patients.[7]

---

[7] Joel Huovian, Sami Kastien, Simo Komulainen, Vasilelos Katsaros, et al. Journal of Neurological Sciences

7. June 2018- Identical Twins with Idiopathic Normal Pressure Hydrocephalus

This case study is from Sweden. Cardiovascular risk factors and subsequent vascular disease may contribute to the development of iNPH. There are data of familial clusters of iNPH suggesting at least some kind of genetic influence or propensity for developing iNPH. [8]

---

[8] Andreas Eleftheriou and Fredik Lundin Journal of Neurological Disorders

8. <u>December 2023- Cases of familial idiopathic normal pressure hydrocephalus implicate genetic factors in disease pathogenesis</u>

There are currently no idiopathic normal pressure hydrocephalus disease genes or biomarkers. In this 2 part analysis, we review literature-based evidence for inheritance of idiopathic normal pressure hydrocephalus in 22 pedigrees, and then present a novel case series of 8 familial iNPH patients. All novel familial NPH patients exhibited improvement following shunt treatment and absence of neurodegenerative cortical pathology, in contrast to many sporadic cases of iNPH with variable clinical responses.[9]

---

[9] Greenberg ABW, Mehta, NH, Mekbib,KY et al Cerebral Cortex. Volume 33, Issue 23.

Appendix 7

Chronological List: Case Reports Genetic Factors and Familial NPH

1. **February 2011- <u>Segmental copy number loss of SFMBT1 gene in elderly individuals with ventriculomegaly: (Japan)</u>**

   A case study of 1.5% of elderly individuals living in a Japanese community who showed ventriculomegaly with features of iNPH on MRI, which may represent a preclinical stage of iNPH. Among several genetic changes observed, a copy number loss with the SFMBT1 gene was seen in half of the ventriculomegaly cases, That was rare among Japanese control subjects.[10]

2. **<u>2016-The SFMBT1 gene is a genetic risk for Shunt-Responsive iNPH</u>**

This case study examined the SFMBT1 gene in patients with shunt-responsive iNPH, healthy elderly and segmental copy of the gene was more frequently observed in the iNPH Disease patients. Therefore, the alteration in the gene may be a genetic risk for iNPH.[11]

---

[10] Kato T, Sato H, Emi M, Seini T, Arawaka S, Iseki C, et al

Internal Medicine

[11] Hidenori S, Yoshimi T, Luna K, Chifumi I, Haiime K, Suzuki, Ryosuke I, Hiroyasu S, et al.

Journal.pon

3. December 2018- <u>Copy number loss in SFMBT1 is common among Finnish and Norwegian patients with iNPH (Finland and Norway)</u>

This is the largest and the first multinational study reporting the increased prevalence of the copy number loss in intron 2 of SFMBT1 among patients with iNPH, providing further evidence of its role in iNPH. 560 Finnish with iNPH and 377 Norwegian patients with iNPH were compared with 508 Finnish elderly, neurologically healthy controls. The copy number loss in intron loss of SFMBT1 was detected in 10% of

Finnish and in 21% of Norwegian patients with iNPH compared to 5.4% in Finnish controls.[12]

4.2019-Prevalence of C90RF72 Expansion in a Large Series of Patients with iNPH (Finland)

This is the first study cohort identifying the underlying C9ORF72 expansion in patients with iNPH. Analysis of the C90RF72 expansion should be considered for patients with probable iNPH presenting with frontal atrophy and severe psychiatric symptoms.[13]

---

[12] Korhonen VE, Helisalmi S, Jokinen A, I Lehtola JM, Oinas M.et al. Neuro Genet 2018

[13] Ville Korhonen et al. Dement Geriatr Cogn Disorder

5. April 2019-Nonsense Mutation in CFAP43 Causes Normal Pressure Hydrocephalus with Ciliary Abnormalities (Japan)

A Japanese study was published in Neurology magazine in 2019. The goal was to identify genes associated with NPH in a Japanese family with several members who had NPH. It identified a loss of function CFAP43 mutation that is most likely responsible for the disease in this family.

The proband was a Japanese woman who was diagnosed with NPH along with a brother, her mother, and another brother who showed significant signs of NPH.

The study obtained genomic DNA samples from the proband, the brothers who was diagnosed with NPH and 3 other siblings who did not develop the disease.

This study generated CFAP43 knockout mice. The brains of these knockout mice were examined to detect signs of hydrocephalus. The CFAP43 knockout mice developed hydrocephalus.[14]

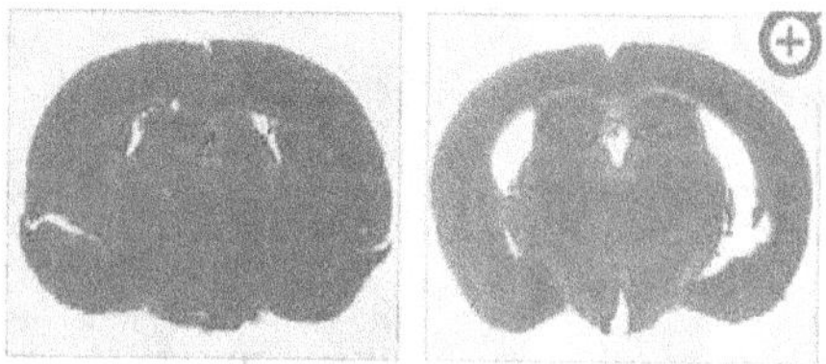

Figure 47: The knockout mouse's brain shows dilatation of the third and lateral ventricles 4/2019

---

[14] Yoshiro Morimoto, Shintaro Yoshida, Akira Kinoshita, Chisel Satah, et al. Neurology Magazine

6. March 2022 -Epidemiology of Idiopathic Normal Pressure Hydrocephalus and Hereditary Hydrocephalus (Japan)

Several genes associated with congenital hydrocephalus have been found, including ciliopathy-related genes that directly affect the ependymal cilia in ventricles. Loss of the copy number of SFMBT1 was found to be a risk factor for iNPH. Knowledge about risk genes and their mechanisms in congenital and familial NPH may be a clue for the further understanding of iNPH. It assumes that less than 10% of patients with iNPH are referred to hospitals in Japan.[15]

---

[15] Chifumi Iseki, Department of Neurology and Clinical Neuroscience, Faculty of Medicine, Yamagata University

7. October 2023-PCWH43 Variants Are Associated with Disease Risk and Clinical Phenotypic Measures in Patients with Normal Pressure Hydrocephalus (United States)

There is growing evidence that variants in specific genes may contribute to NPH. Variants in several genes have been associated with the NPH phenotype including SFMBT1, DNAH14, CFAP43, and CWH43. Predicted loss-of-function mutations were the most common with CWH43. Our findings suggest that congenital factors, rather than malabsorption or vascular dysfunction, are primary contributors to the CWH43 related NPH clinical syndrome.[16]

---

[16] Philip Tipton, MD, Merve Atik MD, Alexandra I. Soto-Beasley, MS. Gregory S. Day, et al. Neurol Genetics

8. December 2023-A Role for Mutations in AK9 and other genes affecting ependymal cells in Normal Pressure Hydrocephalus (United States)

Here, they identify mutations affecting nine additional genes (AK9, RXFP2, PRKD1, HAVCR1, OTOG MYO7A, NOTCH1, SPG11, and MYH13) that are statistically enriched among iNPH patients. The encoded proteins are all highly expressed in choroid plexus and ependymal cells, and most have been associated with cilia. Damaging mutations in AK9 were detected in 9.6% of iNPH patients. Our findings suggest that heterozygous mutations that impair ventricular function may contribute to iNPH.[17]

---

[17] Hong Wei Yang, Semin Lee, Betheny C. Berry, Dejun Yang, Shaokuan Zheng, Rona S. Carroll, Peter J. Park, Mark D. Johnson Proc National Academy Sciences U.S.

9. <u>September 2024-Groundbreaking study uncovers new genetic variants linked to normal pressure hydrocephalus (Finland)</u>

A new study by the University of Eastern Finland and partners identified new genetic variants associated with NPH. The idiopathic form of NPH has been observed to occur in families to some extent, and previous genetic studies have identified individual variants that increase the risk of NPH. The genome-wide association study included 1,522 NPH patients and over 450,000 controls. The study identified significant variants associated with NPH in six different loci. The newly identified gene loci provide a biological relevant foundation for further investigations into disease mechanisms in NPH. Some of these genes have previously been found to associate with the structures or functions of brain areas significant for NPH. Up to 20% of patients with iNPH have at least 1 relative with possible or probable iNPH. One gene SLCO1A2 in the microvascular system is intriguing given the heavy burden of vascular comorbidities of NPH. This is the largest genome-wide assoc. study in the world.[18]

---

[18] Joel Rasanen, Sami Heikkinen, Klira Maklin, Anssi Lipponen, Teemu Kuulasmaa, Juha Mehtonen, Ville E. Korhonen and Ville Leinonon

University of Eastern Finland, Neurology

Appendix 8

Other Imaging Tools

1. APV Index or ALVI-

   A measurement of the ventricles, the APV Index or ALVI "Anteroposterior Diameter of the Lateral Ventricles Index" is calculated by dividing the anteroposterior diameter of the lateral ventricles by the maximum inner skull diameter at the same level on an axial image. Some studies suggest ALVI may be a better indicator for NPH diagnosis as it more accurately reflects ventricular volume.

2. Splenial Angle-

   Another measurement that is rather new is the Splenial Angle. It is used particularly on axial

MRI images . It helps differentiate between iNPH and other conditions like Alzheimer's and Parkinson's disease.

3. Cisternogram-

   Another diagnostic test is the cisternogram. Again, this is for MRI scans and is typically used when the diagnosis is uncertain like maybe the interpretation of the lumbar puncture. The test helps confirm NPH by detecting impaired CSF dynamics, often showing delayed clearance or reflux of radiotracer into the ventricles. It's particularly useful in distinguishing NPH from other conditions like Alzheimer's or vascular dementia.

Appendix 9

Poland Review Article 2024

Normal Pressure Hydrocephalus is a neurological condition that often goes misdiagnosed, leading to significant challenges for those affected. With symptoms that overlap with various types of dementia and Parkinson's disease, NPH remains a critical area of interest within the medical community. In Poland, as in many other countries, the diagnosis and treatment of NPH present unique challenges and opportunities.

In Poland, it is estimated that a significant portion of the elderly population suffers from undiagnosed NPH. Studies suggest that up to 10 percent of nursing home residents may have NPH, yet only a fraction receive the correct diagnosis. This discrepancy is a result of the condition's subtle and overlapping symptoms, which include cognitive decline, gait disturbances, and urinary incontinence. These symptoms mimic other neurological symptoms making accurate diagnosis challenging. In Poland, healthcare providers are encouraged to consider NPH in patients presenting with these symptoms, especially when there is a rapid progression of the disease.

One of the key factors in distinguishing NPH from other dementias is the responsiveness to cerebrospinal fluid (CSF) drainage. In clinical settings, a significant improvement in symptoms following a lumbar puncture can strongly indicate NPH. However, such procedures are not routine and can be overlooked, leading to misdiagnosis.

While NPH is predominantly seen as a sporadic condition, there is ongoing research into potential genetic factors. Studies conducted in Poland have begun to explore familial patterns and genetic predispositions to NPH. Although these studies are in the early stages, they hold promise for future diagnostic and therapeutic approaches.

The primary treatment for NPH involves the surgical insertion of a shunt to drain excess CSF from the brain. In Poland, neurosurgical centers have reported varying degrees of success with shunt surgeries. The clinical outcomes are generally positive, with many patients experiencing significant improvements in gait and cognitive function.

However, the decision to proceed with surgery is complex and requires careful evaluation of potential risks and benefits. In Poland, as elsewhere, there is a need for standardized protocols to guide the treatment of NPH, ensuring that patients receive the best possible care.

Raising awareness about NPH is crucial in improving diagnosis and treatment rates. In Poland, public health campaigns and educational initiatives are essential to inform both healthcare providers and the general public about this condition. Greater awareness can lead to earlier diagnosis and intervention, improving the quality of life for those affected.

Here is a link to the entire research article.

Normal Pressure Hydrocephalus, or Hakim syndrome: review and update[19]

---

[19] Philip W. Tipton, Benjamin D. Elder, Petrice M. Cogswell, Neill Graff-Radford, Department of Neurology, Mayo Clinic, Jacksonville, Florida, US, Department of Neurosurgery, Mayo Clinic, Rochester, Minnesota Copyright 2024 Polis

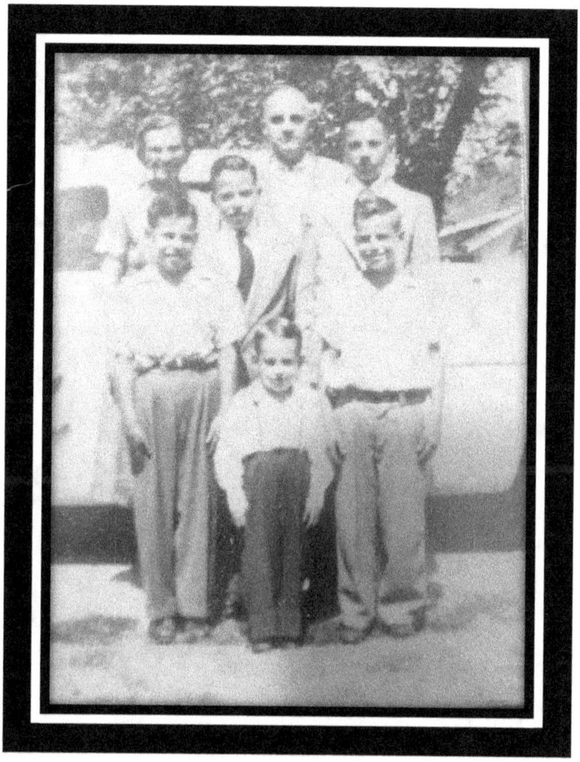

The Shunt Brother's Circa 1950's

Author's Contact E-Mail: doreen0300@att.net

www.ingramcontent.com/pod-product-compliance
Lightning Source LLC
LaVergne TN
LVHW052227200926
848481LV00001B/229